RECLAIM YOUR GUT

AN AUTOIMMUNE PROTOCOL TO STOP LEAKY GUT,
INFLAMMATORY BOWEL DISEASE, AND SIBO USING
A SIMPLE FIVE STEP PLAN

DR. STRONG DC DACNB CFMP PAK

CONTENTS

<u>SPECIAL BONUS!</u>

Want This Bonus Book and A 30-Day Meal Plan for <u>FREE</u>?

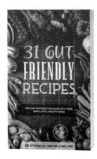 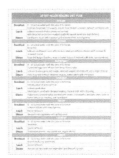

Get <u>FREE</u>, unlimited access to these and all of our new books by joining our community!

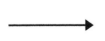

Scan w/ your camera To JOIN!

INTRODUCTION

The greatest trait of humans is that no one individual is alike. Even though we are genetically quite similar, our biochemistry can vary vastly. Why does this matter? Let me explain, there are some of you who have been struggling to maintain good health their entire lives, and that is due to chronic conditions, or lifestyle choices, or both. These symptoms make your life uncomfortable, and these symptoms can make each day a struggle. You may be experiencing chronic fatigue, weight gain, pain, bloating, bouts of gas, acne, insomnia, depression, and anxiety. All of these symptoms are common, debilitating, and can be damaging to your physical *and* emotional health. It's hard to be self-confident and happy on a daily basis when each day is filled with pain and discomfort.

With this book, not only will you establish a solution to your problems, but it will also guide you through a few simple steps to change your lifestyle and reduce the damaging effects of those symptoms. This will make you more confident and positively affect your mental health. This book can resolve your health issues, if you let it! It's filled with tested solutions that can usher in life-changing benefits through smart testing. If you have been looking for a step-by-step guide to reclaiming your health and understanding the gut, then this is it. With the methods found in this book, you can effectively alleviate any external factors that are deteriorating your lifestyle and help you live the life of health and normalcy you desire.

My name is Dr. Strong, and I am a functional medicine practitioner who has worked with hundreds of patients over the years. My patients have complained to me about everything under the sun, from chronic fatigue, pain, migraines, and autoimmune issues, to unexpected weight gain. I have worked with them hand-in-hand and supported them on their path to a better quality of life. My intentions for this book are to be a facilitator and walk this path with you — just like I have with them. When I was younger, I struggled to establish a tangible definition of what health meant. My diet was awful, and the constant thought of my health concerns limited my ability to enjoy life. My desire to understand this led me to my career as a medical practitioner. My goal now is to provide you with the education and motivation to face your health-related problems head-on. I want you to use the knowledge in this book to take control and resolve your health issues once and for all. It's my life's mission to show as many people as possible that information and motivation are the keys to a happy and healthy life.

This book uses a contemporary approach to identifying what is causing internal issues and is designed to help you create a unique lifestyle that optimizes your health, giving you the tools to live the way you have always dreamed of. Chronic fatigue, pain, weight gain, bloating, depression, and anxiety aren't problems that you are stuck with forever. It is time to take control of your health NOW! These health issues are holding you back from your true potential. Do not let them be a deterrent toward the success you are capable of!

Patients who follow my protocols often thank me for changing their lives. They are no longer tormented by the chronic health issues their lives revolved around. It's time to take an active stand for your health using the training that I have listed here. Becoming a healthy individual isn't hard, as long as you have the drive, determination, and will to succeed. With my help and expertise, you will have the know-how to make the transition from struggling through daily life to becoming a thriving, healthy human being.

Take a moment and imagine yourself waking up without your symptoms. What would that kind of day feel like? What kinds of conversations would you have? What would that allow you to do? Visualize it and embrace it — this book is the key to that future.

Your lifestyle is built on a foundation of habits. "Old habits die hard" is stubbornly true — especially when it comes to your health. But by staying on your current path associated with regularly occurring health issues, the chances of you developing a chronic disease only increases. When you decided to read this book, you took the first step to taking back the ownership of your life and reducing your risk of developing future diseases. Remember, your health is *the* most important asset that you can invest in. The longer you wait, the harder it gets. This is why you must take this step towards regaining your life back now, because any delay could lead to disease. Do not let that happen.

As we move through these chapters together, you will find gut-healing information, protocols, and supplements that have yielded positive, beneficial, and repeatable results for everyone that has used them. Every chapter in the book provides you with actionable steps to empower you to get rid of gut issues, undesirable habits, and any other behaviors holding you back. My advice is to treat this book as an interactive guide. Try and form new habits and implement my advice as you read the book. Your life can be longer, healthier, and happier if you commit. Following each of these protocols is your best shot at never dealing with gut issues again.

At this point, you might think there is not enough proof to justify my statements, so I think it's time to show you a patient testimonial. This testimonial is from a patient that I have walked a personal journey with, and I think you will find her story inspiring.

"I was dealing with neck pain on and off for some time. It was suggested that I see Dr. Todd Strong and find out if he could help me resolve my pain, just as he did for a friend of mine. He adjusted me and used a different approach than I was familiar with from past chiropractors, but I finally found something that worked. My pain was gone and didn't return; it was like magic!"

"I told Dr. Strong that I have had Multiple Sclerosis (MS) for 13 years and experience constant issues with walking and falling. My legs would give out, rendering me helpless for periods of time. This made it difficult to go out in public with confidence because of the fear of what people would think. I had been on several different medications with no results and tried many alternative methods that were costly to try to

alleviate symptoms. Some worked for a little while, but my symptoms would always come back. Dr. Strong explained the importance of gut and brain health, and he suggested I start a cleanse for my gut, followed by a liver detox."

"It was weeks of clean eating and understanding what I was putting in my body. It was hard at first, but it gave me a chance to improve my quality of life with food and not medicine. I noticed a difference shortly after and haven't fallen or had trouble walking ever since! I am truly grateful that I came across a doctor that practices functional medicine and had the knowledge to know how to treat my symptoms with success. It's been 13 years living with Multiple Sclerosis and to be able to live without the embarrassment and concern of not knowing if I can get up and walk without falling is PRICELESS."
"I tell everyone about what helped me and wouldn't be where I am with my health without the knowledge and insight of Dr. Todd Strong. Thank you!"

The people I work with have health concerns that often fall through the cracks of standard medications and surgery. These people care about their bodies and have a desire to change, but they have hit dead end after dead end. As it turned out, all they needed was a little guidance. When these people are given a chance to turn their lives around, they grab the opportunity with both hands. If you were to ask anyone that I have helped and whether or not the journey that they went on was easy, they would probably tell you it was not. However, when we are pushed to our limits and challenged, we appreciate the value of our struggles. They have done it, and now it is your turn to do the same.

1

AN INTRODUCTION TO GUT HEALTH: WHAT YOU NEED TO KNOW

Our gut plays a major role within our bodies. It handles the absorption of essential vitamins, minerals, and the removal of waste products. Think of it like a filtration system. It takes out what we need from the foods we eat, absorbs them, and then filters out what our bodies don't need.

Dysfunction in how your gut absorbs nutrients and removes waste products can cause a great deal of harm to the body. An example of this would be amino acids. Amino acids are obtained from protein and are essential in neurotransmitter production, muscle repair, bone reconstruction, and strengthening. If you cannot get the right amount of amino acids due to a defect in your gut (resulting in a term that we call 'malabsorption'), you cannot carry out any of these processes. This directly impacts your daily life, as you are unable to adequately produce neurotransmitters (depression/anxiety), repair muscle (soreness), and reinforce your bone (fractures). Another common example is iron. Iron acts in our blood by allowing oxygen to be effectively transported around the body, supplying our tissues and muscles with the substances needed to perform their functions effectively. When someone has the inability to absorb iron effectively, we say that the person is *anemic*. If iron malabsorption is due to an unhealthy gut, you can eliminate any inkling of anemia that was present or that may develop in the future by rectifying your gut health.

When our gut doesn't function correctly, we develop specific signs and symptoms that can alert ourselves and healthcare practitioners of dysfunction in the body. When looking at the complexity of the gut, several varying symptoms and signs present themselves. Some of these signs and symptoms include the following:

- **An upset stomach:** Disturbances felt in your stomach, or any other part of the gut, may make you feel like your stomach is full of gas, giving rise to the feeling of being bloated. This can also be combined with constipation or diarrhea. Even heartburn can be a sign of an unhealthy gut. When we compare this to a balanced and healthy gut, there is less difficulty processing food and eliminating waste products.

- **Sugar cravings:** Our guts contain between 300 to 500 different types of bacteria, with many of the bacteria being termed 'good' bacteria, contributing to the smooth functioning of our bodies. However, a diet that is high in processed foods and sugars will destroy and diminish the number of good bacteria in your gut. This imbalance creates a craving for sugar-rich foods, further damaging your gut. High amounts of refined sugars, like corn syrup that exhibit elevated levels of fructose, have also been shown to increase the degree of inflammation that the body experiences.

- **Unintentional changes in weight:** We expect weight change when trying a new exercise regimen or an altered diet, but if you are gaining or losing weight without these changes, it is a sign that an unhealthy gut is developing. An imbalanced gut impairs your body's ability to absorb nutrients, store fat, and regulate blood sugar levels. It can even lead to instances of small intestinal bacterial overgrowth (SIBO) if weight loss is occurring or increased insulin resistance if you are gaining weight.

- **A sense of constant fatigue with or without sleep disturbances:** Having an unhealthy gut contributes to sleep disturbances like insomnia and poor sleep. If left unchecked, these gut problems can lead to chronic fatigue as well. Your gut produces the majority of your serotonin (a hormone that affects your mood and sleep patterns), so if you damage your gut, you are risking a negative impact to your ability to sleep well.

- **Skin irritation:** Eczema has been linked to a damaged gut. Gut inflammation causes an increase in the 'leaking' out of proteins from your body. These proteins irritate the skin in such a way that it presents as having eczema. Many people think that they have a skin condition, which they technically do, but this symptom is secondary to the underlying root of the problem, your gut health.

- **Autoimmune conditions:** Research is still ongoing within this field, but the results thus far show a favorable link between the direct impact an unhealthy gut has on the presence of inflammation in the body and the overall functioning of our immune system. This can lead to autoimmune responses, which is when the body attacks itself instead of the foreign organisms that may have found their way into our bodies. Coupled with stress, this is a dangerous recipe for disaster.

- **Food intolerances:** An intolerance is the inability to digest certain foods, and that's different from a food allergy. A food allergy is the body's immune response to certain foods, which can show varying reactions including anaphylaxis (in severe cases) or a small bout of diarrhea (minor cases). Some studies have linked low quality of bacteria in guts to food intolerances, and the most frequent symptoms are bloating, increased gas or flatulence, diarrhea, nausea, and abdominal pain.

Many of the instances above are treated as acute (i.e. having a sudden onset that is resolved when the problem is removed) however, if an acute problem isn't identified and treated quickly, living with it could progress into a chronic condition. Chronic conditions tend to require lifelong therapy, leading to more complicated health conditions. They often require you to take varying amounts of medications, which may further irritate your gut. This creates a compounding effect and is what this book is helping you prevent. Here are a few of the chronic conditions you can avoid by keeping your gut healthy, and we also dive into the details of these in subsequent chapters.

- **Small intestinal bacterial overgrowth (SIBO):** SIBO is a serious healthcare condition that occurs when bacteria that are usually localized to a particular area in the gut start to grow in other areas of the small intestine. These bacteria do not belong there, and this misplacement often causes pain and diarrhea. Bacteria eat to survive like any other organism. They use up the nutrients that we ingest as their energy source, resulting in a lot less of the essential vitamins and minerals being used by the body. The more bacteria that are present, the more nutrients will be consumed. This results in a diminished supply of nutrients for the body to utilize. A list of common symptoms include stomach pain (especially after eating), bloating, cramps, diarrhea, constipation, indigestion, a constant feeling of fullness, and an increased amount of gas being produced. These symptoms are caused by bacteria affecting the pH levels in the small intestine and gut, resulting in small intestine malfunctions. SIBO is also associated with an array of other gut-based conditions such as viral gastroenteritis (typically known and caused by the stomach bug) and celiac disease. Don't worry, SIBO is easily treated with a combination of herbal supplements and diet change. However, some cases may warrant more extensive measures.

- **Leaky gut syndrome (LGS):** LGS is a condition of the gut that affects the lining of the intestines. It is exactly what its name implies — irritants widen gaps in between the intestinal wall, allowing bacteria and other toxins to pass into the bloodstream. Our body tags these newcomers as foreign bodies, creating an immune response of marked inflammation. It is this inflammation in combination with fatigue, headaches, chronic diarrhea, constipation, bloating, or skin problems such as eczema that point healthcare professionals toward diagnosing a patient with LGS. It's worth noting that your chances of developing LGS increase when you have a pre-existing chronic condition, so people who suffer from diabetes, lupus, and chronic strength deficits should pay special attention to their gut health.

- **Irritable bowel syndrome (IBS):** Commonly affecting the large intestine, IBS is a chronic condition that needs long-term management. IBS includes abdominal pain, cramping, and bloating that seems to be relieved after a bowel movement. This is usually seen with excessive gas production, alternating bouts of diarrhea and constipation, and occasional presence of mucus in the stool. Gut health is the core factor when ensuring IBS does not occur. This is because poor gut health can result in inflammation of the intestines, a severe infection, changes in bacteria, and gut microflora, which are all risk factors for IBS development. IBS can also be triggered by food, hormones, and even high levels of stress.

- **Celiac disease:** The disease that made the gluten-free diet famous, this condition is an autoimmune disease of genetic and environmental origin where the ingestion of gluten causes damage to the small intestine. The main area of attack is the lining of your small intestine, which inhibits the effective absorption of nutrients. This condition has a genetic predisposition, and if left untreated it can lead to other autoimmune diseases, such as, type 1 diabetes and multiple sclerosis (MS). Treatment includes adherence to a strict gluten-free diet, which encompasses avoiding wheat, barley, rye, bread, and beer. Celiac disease has generic symptoms such as vomiting, diarrhea, constipation and fatigue. However, the unique symptoms to this condition include the development of attention deficit hyperactivity disorder (ADHD), a short stature, iron-deficiency anemia, pale, foul-smelling, or fatty stools, and even dental enamel defects of permanent teeth.

- **Gastroesophageal reflux disease (GERD):** Your gut runs from your mouth to the anus, in other words, from the point of entry to the point of exit. GERD is a digestive disorder where stomach juices and fluids move back up from the stomach into the esophagus. Symptoms include difficulty or pain when swallowing, acid regurgitation (best described as tasting your food again after eating it), inflammation of your gums, bad breath, and constantly present laryngitis or hoarseness. When juices from your stomach repeatedly enter your esophagus, the lining of the esophagus is damaged, leading to additional healthcare problems. As the cells in your esophagus change due to the constant acid exposure, foods that were easy to eat before may be difficult to consume. GERD is best prevented through weight loss, decreasing alcohol intake, and limiting meal sizes. These changes significantly reduce the risk of chronic complications and incidence rate of GERD.

Many of the conditions I have listed all begin with an unhealthy gut. Maintaining our gut health is important if we want to experience a life of health and happiness, but what if some of the damage is already done? What can we do to start rectifying our current gut health? Here are a few options we have:

- **Starting on a probiotic to re-establish the correct levels of 'good' bacteria in your gut.** This will decrease the types of bacteria that are directly related to poor gut health, lower the chances of contracting infections, and have an evident impact on your immediate health.

- **Changing your diet,** especially if you are aware of food intolerances but continue to eat those foods anyway. The substances you are intolerant toward are toxic for your body. They are killing you slowly and doing a lot more harm than good.

- **Reducing stress.** Stress is a broad term that includes psychological stress, environmental stress, sleep deprivation, and the disruption of the circadian rhythm (the cycle that we go through when sleeping). Do not underestimate how much of an effect stress has on the body. Stress is widely damaging and can directly affect the health of your gut, so we must keep this in mind when planning our path toward a healthy gut.

By starting with these achievable lifestyle changes, I guarantee you will feel a difference. As we move forward in this book, remember that everyone is different and that some people can tolerate certain foods that others can't. Ultimately, the gut is where all of your vitamins and minerals are absorbed. Without a healthy gut, you are unable to absorb the resources that fuel your body and allow it to function optimally — whatever optimal may mean to you.

2

AUTOIMMUNITY: A WAR ZONE IN YOUR BODY

The body is a complicated machine. There are so many factors that need to be taken into consideration when we look at what the "normal" functioning of the human body entails. This chapter aims to equip you with the basic biology you need to know about your body and how that relates to your gut health. By developing a basic understanding of how your body works, you can understand why some conditions happen when they do, including why they cause specific symptoms. We will look at how proteins, bacteria, environmental toxins, and other pathogens (disease-causing microorganisms) can leak through the gut, traverse its natural barriers, and enter the bloodstream. When the body recognizes these pathogens, it attacks itself, leading to chronic inflammation, pain, brain fog (a loss in the ability to think clearly), depression, anxiety, and weight gain. The healing of an unhealthy gut will eliminate these symptoms.

Autoimmunity is a term we hear a lot, especially in the context of pre-existing conditions, and you may have wondered what it really is. *Autoimmunity is the process of your body fighting against itself.* It identifies its own cells as foreign, attacking them in an attempt to establish a sense of equilibrium. This happens most often when a site-specific group of cells is found in an area in which they do not belong. An example would be bacteria that have leaked into the bloodstream via inflamed pores in the gut. Bacteria does not belong here, and the body will react to their presence by attempting to destroy them. Think of your immune system as a security guard, allowing only approved cells in specific areas to pass while removing any that shouldn't.

The process of autoimmunity results in the possible causation of autoimmune diseases. An autoimmune disease is a condition that follows the same mechanism as above. The body's immune system cannot tell the difference between the foreign cells that have infiltrated the body and normal, healthy cells. More specifically, the immune system can mistake a part of your body, like your joints and skin, as foreign. This results in a release of proteins called auto-antibodies that attack healthy cells. Some autoimmune diseases are restricted to one specific organ, like type 1 diabetes that damages the pancreas, and others like systemic lupus erythe-matous (SLE) that attack the whole body.

Researchers have been working hard to identify the environmental factors that may cause autoimmune diseases, and they found that adopting a western diet resulted in a drastic decrease in the health of a person's gut. A typical western diet set off a cascade of inflammatory responses due to the presence of high-fat, high-sugar, and processed foods being ingested. This demonstrates a direct correlation between diet and autoimmune responses, due to irritants that diminish organ protection barriers and/or ingested toxins that follow the same mechanism.

Here's an extensive list of autoimmune diseases that may be caused by poor diet and gut health:

- **Type 1 diabetes:** This condition is primarily due to the dysfunction of the pancreas, an organ responsible for the production of the hormones insulin, glucagon, and somatostatin. Insulin is the hormone that is responsible for regulating blood sugar levels in the body. However, in type 1 diabetes, the immune system attacks the pancreas, destroying the insulin-producing cells (also known as the beta cells) in the pancreas. This results in high blood sugar levels that cause a condition called hyperglycemia, which can lead to blood vessel damage and possibly injure the heart, kidneys, eyes, and nerves. The actions of insulin and glucagon work together. When there is too much sugar present in the bloodstream, insulin is released to lower it. When there is too little sugar in the bloodstream, glucagon will be released to elevate the sugar concentration in the bloodstream. It is in this way that a sugar balance is established in our bodies.

- **Rheumatoid arthritis (RA):** With this condition, the body's joints are attacked by the body's immune system. This causes redness, warmth, and feelings of stiffness in the joints. RA can begin as young as 30 years old, which is why it is important to monitor your gut health from an early age. The usual treatments for RA feature long-term medication that may alter the defense mechanisms of your body, leading to an increased risk of infections and a direct impact on your ability to live a healthy and active lifestyle. To ensure that these domino effects are avoided, you must maintain adequate gut health.

- **Psoriasis:** Our skin cells work by using a shedding mechanism. When the skin cells have grown and are no longer needed, we shed. In psoriasis, the skin cells multiply too quickly, and this excess of cells forms red inflamed patches that look like a pattern of silver-white scales traversing over the skin. Due to the constant presence of inflammation in this condition, if it remains untreated, it can progress to an arthritic form of psoriasis, causing joint swelling, stiffness, and pain.

- **Multiple sclerosis (MS):** Having an unhealthy gut damages both body cells and nerve cells. There is a part of the nerve called the myelin sheath that conducts impulses from your brain down to your muscles, allowing you to move your body. With an unhealthy gut, the myelin sheath can be damaged, which drastically slows down the relayed messages between your brain, spinal cord, and the rest of your body. This damage can result in numbness, weakness, balance issues, and even impact your ability to walk.

- **Systemic lupus erythematosus (SLE):** A skin disease where an unhealthy gut causes your body to attack its own healthy tissue and results in rashes around organs, joints, brain, heart, and kidneys. SLE is commonly identified by the 'butterfly rash' that forms across the face. When comparing SLE condition to other autoimmune diseases caused by an unhealthy gut, we can see how an unhealthy gut impacts the entire body and not just a specific segment.

- **Inflammatory bowel disease:** We have already established that an unhealthy gut produces toxins that affect the lining of the intestinal wall, making the absorption of vitamins and minerals difficult. Depending on where the inflammation occurs, the form of inflammatory bowel disease is named differently. Crohn's disease is inflammation anywhere from the mouth to the anus, and ulcerative colitis is specifically related to the large intestine and rectum lining.

- **Addison's disease:** When an unhealthy gut affects the kidneys, there is a direct impact on the adrenal glands that are attached on top of the kidneys. The adrenal glands produce the hormones cortisol and aldosterone. Having too little cortisol affects how the body stores carbohydrates and glucose, causing excessive sodium loss and excess potassium in the bloodstream. This in turn exacerbates the mineral imbalance that was initially caused by the unhealthy gut. Addison's disease symptoms include bouts of weakness, fatigue, low blood sugar, and weight loss. Cortisol is also the hormone released in response to stress, whether it be environmental or emotional. We discuss cortisol in detail in a later chapter.

- **Myasthenia gravis:** When an unhealthy gut affects the nerves, the impulses that help the brain control your muscles are affected. When these nerve conduction pathways are impaired, the muscles cannot receive adequate signals to contract, resulting in a condition called "myasthenia gravis." A common symptom is muscle weakness that gets progressively worse with continued activity, with strength returning to normal after rest. The muscles affected can be broad, though, extending to the muscles in our face and resulting in abnormal control of eye movements, eyelid opening, and swallowing.

- **Pernicious anemia:** When the stomach lining is harmed due to an unhealthy gut, a deficiency in a protein known as *intrinsic factor (IF)* occurs. This protein is necessary for vitamin B12 absorption from food, affecting the body's ability to undergo DNA synthesis. Untreated pernicious anemia can cause heart and nerve damage.

- **Hashimoto's Disease:** This is when toxins, potentially produced by an unhealthy gut, migrate to the thyroid gland in the neck, causing an immune response to occur. From here, the thyroid becomes damaged and unable to function properly. Since the thyroid is responsible for regulating your metabolism, proper hormone function, proper neural and musculoskeletal development, this can lead to issues in the aforementioned systems. Common symptoms include weight gain, chronic fatigue, chronic pain/inflammation, and depression. Many thyroid patients that have gut issues as well may be overlooking the root cause of their thyroid issues.

- **Sjögren's syndrome:** An unhealthy gut affects the ability of the glands in the eyes to produce the lubricating agent that ensures that our eyes and mouths do not dry out. When the balance of the body is disturbed, dry eyes and a dry mouth become the hallmark signs of Sjögren's syndrome. This syndrome is proof that an unhealthy gut affects organs that are pivotal in our daily functioning, such as the eyes.

As you can see, the presence of an unhealthy gut can impact different systems and organs in the body through an alarming number of ways. Your nerves, heart, muscle functioning, emotions, and even your degree of metabolism are at risk. I hope that the explanations provided have made you recognize the importance and dramatic effect that gut health has on your life. We have covered the risks, but now we need to talk about *how* and *when* we need to take action. So how do we know when we need to make lifestyle changes to prevent these autoimmune diseases?

The answer to this question depends on your ability to monitor yourself and effectively notice irregularities when they present themselves. Early signs that you might be developing an autoimmune disease include constant fatigue, muscle ache while at rest, red and swollen areas, abnormal hair loss, numbness and tingling in the hands and feet, persistent low-grade fever, and difficulty concentrating. When you start noticing something out of the ordinary, document it so that you have a paper trail of dates and symptoms that you can give to your healthcare professionals. This helps them create a diagnosis faster and treat your condition before it gets out of hand. Remember that some symptoms like redness or swelling come and go, so documenting is the best way to spot patterns that may be indicators of a deeper issue.

Your skin is the largest organ in the human body. Yes, your skin is actually an organ! This is why most people spot skin-related symptoms first, and our skin doesn't just protect our body from the world, it also functions as a detox organ. Sometimes our organs become overloaded and congested, resulting in the skin taking over and pushing toxins from the body out through the skin. Believe it or not, the skin will remove approximately two pounds of waste a day from your body in the form of perspiration. When your body isn't balanced, your skin starts to develop dry spots, eczema, and dark rings under the eyes. How does this relate to an unhealthy gut? If your gut is producing toxins, then that means more toxins will need to be removed from the body, causing your skin to step in and help out the other organs. This is why you should suspect something is off-balance in your body when your skin starts to develop symptoms.

An unhealthy gut is the foundation of chronic diseases, autoimmune issues, and neurological difficulties. All of these secondary effects fall away when you properly address the root cause of the existing problem. The resolution of most of these diseases gives the patient an optimal sense of health. The rate at which this resolution occurs is improved by monitoring your progression and documenting anything unusual that occurred before symptoms began. To prevent your body's tissues from being caught in the crossfire of chronic inflammation and disease, start with the core, and start with your gut.

3

EAT INFLAMMATION, BECOME INFLAMMATION

There are approximately ten times the amount of microorganisms in the gut than somatic (body) cells within the body. The gut is unique because it has 'good' bacteria living alongside yeasts, viruses, and small parasitic worms. Much of this bacteria helps with the fermentation process of undigested food, assisting in the creation of the fecal bulk. When we look at the diet and how it affects the gut, a typical western diet is a precursor for an unhealthy gut. With high levels of carbohydrates, fats, sugars, and protein in western diets, these substrates largely escape digestion and absorption. This occurs in the the small intestine, negatively influencing the effect of bacteria and microorganisms near the end of the gut. With a diet that is high in carbohydrates (specifically refined starches), the development of a large and compact fecal mass is decreased.

FREQUENTLY ASKED QUESTIONS ABOUT COMMON GUT IRRITANTS

Dairy

Why is dairy seen as an irritant to the gut?

The high levels of lactose present in dairy products are what irritate the gut. If your body is unable to digest the excess lactose, you become bloated and start to build up gas, passing it frequently. If you keep ingesting dairy containing products, the lactose interacts with the large intestine's bacteria, resulting in diarrhea and a worsening of bloating and gas production. When your body doesn't have enough of the enzyme lactase (responsible for breaking down lactose), then the lactose gets broken down by bacteria, resulting in the already mentioned symptoms. This is why lactose-intolerant people avoid dairy products — they lack the lactase enzyme. And if left unchecked, permanent damage can occur to the large intestine. Being in a constant state of inflammation from dairy can also negatively affect your ability to operate effectively, get tasks done, and meet personal deadlines.

What are common dairy-containing products?

Since lactose is found primarily in milk, foods that are high in lactose will contain milk. Dishes and single ingredients that contain large amounts of lactose include milk, macaroni and cheese, yogurt, cottage cheese, and most desserts. Some meal supplements are also high in lactose, so it is important to check labels when considering implementing a supplement into your diet.

How much dairy is too much dairy?

When we look at amounts of dairy products that are okay to ingest, we run into a problem. Some individuals can ingest dairy with no symptoms or issues, others may have a minor reaction, such as gas/bloating, and some people may even develop flu-like symptoms. Everyone is different, and assessing your own food sensitivities is crucial to maintaining your health. If you experience gut irritation when using dairy products, all dairy products should be eliminated from your diet.

Is there a difference between good dairy and bad dairy?

Dairy is not classified as healthy or unhealthy. Instead, it is referred to as a 'tolerance potential.' This is because the effect that dairy has on the body varies from person to person, and there is no compelling evidence that shows ingesting dairy products is inherently risky.

What will happen in my gut if I ingest too much dairy?

As the saying goes, "too much of anything is bad for you." Dairy products do contain levels of fat within them, so when you consume too much dairy, it can lead to nausea, stomach cramps, and diarrhea — even if you are not diagnosed as lactose intolerant. These symptoms occur because our bodies are unable to break down the lactose in our bodies fast enough, leading to more being broken down by bacteria during a fermentation process instead of the normal biological process where lactose is broken down by the lactase enzyme.

Soy

What is soy?

Soy is a legume native to Asia that many vegetarians eat to ensure their recommended protein intake is achieved. Soy can be ingested as a whole food or processed food, the least processed form includes soybeans and edamame (immature soybeans). The most common soy products are soy milk and tofu, which are made from whole soybeans. Fermented soy products are processed into soy sauce (a condiment made from fermented soy, salt water, mold, and roasted grains), tempeh (fermented soy cake), and miso (seasoning that includes soybeans, salt, and fungus).

Is soy good for me?

Soy is not good for your body. The soy products that you get at the supermarket are laden with processed preservatives, which destroy any health benefit it would have provided.

With companies like Monsanto, who create genetically modified organisms (GMOs), there is research that shows an increased goitrogenic effect of soy. A goitrogenic effect affects the thyroid's ability to use iodine correctly, which slows down your metabolism. Ultimately, this will make you feel cold and cause you to have a weakened immune system. This, coupled with an unhealthy gut, increases the chances of contracting infections. Soy also contains high amounts of estrogen, which, when taken in high amounts by men, could have detrimental effects on their libido and can promote fat accumulation around the waist. The source of the soy is a very important factor to consider, and depending on where the soy is made, the degree of negative effects that occur will be influenced.

Can I drink soy if I am lactose intolerant?

Yes, you can drink soy milk if you are lactose intolerant. However, I do not recommend drinking soy as an alternative. Depending on the source of the soybeans, soy milk can lead to further health complications. I suggest coconut milk, cashew milk, or another nut milk as a substitute (assuming you aren't allergic).

How does soy cause gut irritation?

Soy is very difficult to digest, so your digestive system tends to rely on gut bacteria to break it down, which causes bloating, gas production, and general discomfort. A study found in the *Journal of Gastroenterology* found that 98% of individuals who regularly included soy in their diet showed a complete halt of bloating and gas production upon removing soy from their daily life. Non-fermented soy is a lot more difficult to digest due to its lack of processing. This is why fermented forms such as the miso and tempeh digest more easily. If you choose to eat soy, try and consume it from fermented sources.

Is soy a good alternative to cow's milk?

No, we recommend using almond milk if you aren't allergic or sensitive to nuts. For nutrient comparison, almond milk is a good source of low-fat and plant-based protein, has less saturated fat than cow's milk, and is also cholesterol-free. Almond milk also has a large number of minerals and vitamins that are necessary for the human body to function optimally.

Corn

How does corn irritate your gut?

Corn is very high in cellulose, which cannot be broken down in a human's digestive system. This leads to the corn undergoing fermentation in the large intestine. The fermented byproducts from the corn, including short-chain fatty acids, hydrogen, carbon dioxide, and methane, lead to a wide array of symptoms that mimic gut irritation, including gas formation, bloating, and diarrhea. If a large amount of corn is ingested, the pressure difference created in the gut due to the byproducts of the fermentation process can result in responses that could be detrimental to your health. This is especially true if corn is combined with other products that have a high chance of fermenting.

How much corn should I be eating?

Corn is high in carbohydrates, fiber, vitamins, and minerals. It's also relatively low in protein and fat, which makes it a good substitute for other carbohydrate-rich foods that you may not enjoy. However, you should eat corn in moderation as its cellulose presence can spark intense gastric symptoms due to its typically genetically modified nature.

What disadvantages are there to eating corn?

Corn, especially corn fructose syrups, contain high concentrations of processed sugars that are detrimental to gut health. Corn undergoes intense levels of genetic modification, decreasing its natural nutrient capabilities. Most GMO foods negatively impact gut health based on their conditions of growth and the degree to which they are genetically modified. With some of the byproducts of GMOs remaining unstudied in the human population, we are not aware of the long-term effects that GMO products can cause. This is why we advocate that GMOs should be avoided whenever possible.

Sugar

Why is sugar seen as a gut irritant?

Sugar contributes to inflammation, a core component of an unhealthy gut. When it isn't impacting inflammation, it destroys the good bacteria present within your gut, which weakens your body's ability to break down foods. Sugar is doubly dangerous because it contributes to weight gain, and if not quickly resolved, a high-sugar diet can cause dietary-induced diabetes that further exacerbates the gut irritant effect of sugars. When you are choosing foods for your diet, or even for your enjoyment, check the nutritional information label for hidden sugars. It is this combination of 'known' sugar and hidden sugars that can exacerbate inflammation.

How much sugar is too much?

The American Heart Association (AHA) recommends that men should not consume more than nine teaspoons of added sugar per day. This equates to roughly 36 grams or 150 calories. For women, however, this value is lower, with a recommended daily intake of six teaspoons of added sugar per day. This equates to roughly 25 grams or 100 calories. To put this in perspective, a single 12-ounce can of soda can contain eight teaspoons of added sugar. The more added sugar you ingest, the higher your risk of gut toxin production, an unhealthy gut, and the development of conditions such as diabetes, atherosclerosis, strokes, and vision and nerve problems.

Will brown sugar affect my gut less negatively than white sugar?

The rule of thumb is that the darker the sugar, the fewer calories and more calcium, iron, and potassium it contains. Because brown sugar is less refined than white sugar, the health benefits are more noticeable. This means that if you were to have one teaspoon over the recommended daily intake, brown sugar would impact your body less negatively due to its decreased calories and well-established mineral profile compared to white sugar.

What different types of sugars are there?

Sugars are more complex than simply the white and brown sugar that you and I know so well. They are divided into simple and complex sugars, and because each different type of sugar serves a unique purpose in the regulation of the body's functioning, they can be found in a variety of different types of foods. Your simple sugars are fructose (found in fruits and honey), galactose (found in milk and dairy products), and glucose (found in honey, fruits, and vegetables). Your simple sugars then combine to form your complex sugars, which are lactose (made from glucose combined with galactose and is found in milk), maltose (made from two glucose molecules in barley), and sucrose (made from glucose combined with fructose found in plants).

Gluten

What does it mean to be gluten-intolerant?

Gluten is a collection of proteins that are found in rye, wheat and barley. When someone is considered gluten-intolerant, they are unable to eat gluten because a person's body will mount an immune response on its own cells, specifically damaging the tiny hair-like projections that line the small intestine. This results in digestive problems that include diarrhea, severe abdominal pain, and excessive gas production.

What are the common gluten-containing foods?

Many processed foods we eat today contain gluten. Some of these include beer, bread, cereals, cookies, croutons, french fries, gravies, pasta, salad dressings, malt, processed lunch meats, and some soup mixes.

How much gluten is too much?

That differs from person to person. In a typical western diet, people can eat 15-30 grams of gluten per day. This amount, while safe for some, can make others really sick. There have been trials attempting to establish a safe threshold of gluten, and these point toward 5 grams as being a healthier threshold. The amount you should eat also depends on whether or not you are on a gluten-free diet (due to gluten intolerance or personal preference), which can range anywhere between 15 and 625 milligrams of gluten per day.

How does gluten cause irritation to the gut?

Gluten activates a substance called zonulin that regulates the permeability of the intestines. When you have too much gluten in your system, a greater amount of zonulin is produced, leading to an increase in the permeability of the intestines (i.e., larger substances can cross between the intestines and the bloodstream). This increased intestinal permeability results in an immune response because the substances crossing the intestine's barrier are recognized as harmful, leading to inflammation.

Are there different types of gluten?

There are two main types of gluten, and they are known as gliadins and glutenins. The gliadins are essential for allowing our baked bread to rise effectively. The glutenin segment causes the swelling of the individual particles to form a continuous network of fine strands that are facilitated by gliadin. These reactions typically occur when water is combined with flour.

Nightshades

What are nightshades?

Nightshade vegetables are part of the *Solanaceae* plant family. Many individuals associate the word 'nightshade' with its toxic brethren known to many as the belladonna plant or deadly nightshade. You may be surprised to find that many of the foods we commonly eat today are a part of the nightshade group. Nightshades contain solanine, an alkaloid substance that is toxic when ingested in high concentrations.

What foods fall into the nightshades group?

Common nightshade vegetables include white potatoes (green potatoes are highly toxic), tomatoes, eggplant, bell peppers, cayenne pepper, and paprika. These vegetables contain trace amounts of solanine, which is why they do not pose a significant health risk when eaten.

How do nightshades cause gut irritation?

Nightshades contain a protein called lectin that damages the intestinal barrier when present in high amounts. This aids in the development of leaky gut syndrome, which causes an inflammatory cascade against foreign bodies that make their way into your bloodstream.

Can you be allergic to nightshades?

Yes, you can. The alkaloid component of the nightshades is what causes the immune response to occur. These allergies can cause breathing problems, a rash, and bouts of eczema shortly after ingesting nightshade vegetables. The extent and severity of the allergic reaction depends on your body's sensitivity to the alkaloid compounds. Symptoms vary from a mild rash and short period of labored breathing to anaphylactic shock.

Hippocrates once said, "let food be thy medicine, and let medicine be thy food." This quote refers to the foundation that stable nutrition and diet afford us. The discussions of the effects of an adequate diet have been studied in great detail across history. In 1903, Thomas Edison was concerned about the healthcare system in his time and stated, "The doctor of the future will give no medicine, but will interest his patient in the care of the human frame, in diet, and in the cause and prevention of disease."

Tracking your diet is one of the best ways to see which foods directly influence your health. This is best achieved with a food diary that records everything you ate up to 12 hours before any symptoms started. Tracking your symptoms this way allows you to recognize patterns and help your health professional with their diagnosis. There are many ways to keep a food journal. You can use a physical journal, take notes in your phone, or use a calendar app. I recommend building your journal into any existing habits you already have. This gives you the best chance at sticking to it.

One of the best tools we have to promote gut health by identifying and eliminating possible irritants is the elimination diet. The elimination diet, which is seen as the gold standard in nutrition circles, cuts out specific types of foods based on the data from your food diary. By comparing before and after results and relating them to your body's health and overall well-being, you can see which foods are negatively affecting your gut.

How the elimination diet is conducted depends on you. Some find it easy to cut everything out of their diet that they know is not good for their health. For others, their body may be so used to the levels of inflammation in their body that by cutting out all foods immediately, their body may crash, making them feel worse than they felt before starting the diet. This is why it's best to work at your own pace, coupled with constant reminders of your end goal — a life rich with health, energy, and peace.

4

ENVIRONMENTAL TOXINS, YOUR ENVIRONMENT, AND YOUR HEALTH

We interact with an array of different environments on a daily basis. Many people work in areas where chemical toxicants are a part of their daily lives, whether they are employed in pest control, the tobacco industry, agriculture, or work in a factory. But what effect do these irritants have on our bodies? How do they affect our gut health? These questions will be answered in this chapter, and we will be focusing on the influence of chemical toxicants, heavy metals, emotional stress, drugs, and the manners and mechanisms in which our health is negatively influenced.

Chemical Toxicants

Chemical toxicants can impact our health in a variety of ways. It is important that we take note of them. If we do not, then they may harm our bodies indefinitely. The degree of our exposure can be the difference between harming our bodies or ensuring a healthy outcome. Here are the major types of chemical toxicants you should be aware of:

- **Aluminium hydroxide as an adjuvant in a vaccine:** An adjuvant is an ingredient that creates a stronger immune response. Vaccines are given to cause an immune response, so these are designed to help vaccines work better. By helping the body produce a strong enough immune response, adjuvants ensure that you are protected against a specific disease. Some vaccines cause local reactions such as redness, swelling, and pain at the injection site, and these are a lot more common in adjuvant vaccines than non-adjuvanted vaccines. Aluminium hydroxide has been used as an adjuvant since the early 1930s. The issue is, the aluminium hydroxide that is used in vaccines is still not very well understood, and the effects are still being studied. What we do know is that if aluminum hydroxide is ingested on its own in large amounts, it causes severe gut pain, muscle weakness, tiredness, bloody stools, and vomit that looks like coffee grounds.

- **Tobacco:** This product is used by smokers as a manner of relaxation and has become ingrained in their daily routines. However, many people aren't aware of the detrimental effect that tobacco has on their gut health. A study compared the types of bacteria found in individuals who smoked versus those who didn't. It found an increase in the *Prevotella* bacteria in individuals that use tobacco. This bacteria is well known in causing an increased risk of colon cancer and inflammation of your large intestine. There was also evidence of a decrease in the *Bacteroides* bacteria in smokers, which are necessary and beneficial probiotics in the body. So apart from the obvious lung and mouth cancer considerations, quitting smoking will also improve your gut health.

- **Glyphosate:** Glyphosate is a herbicide that many who work in fields are exposed to. Constant exposure to this toxicant can result in negative gut-based effects. One of the most prominent effects is the alteration of the pH in the intestines. Our gut (especially our small intestine where absorption of minerals and nutrients takes place) needs to have a regulated pH for adequate intake. However, glyphosate increases the pH of the intestinal contents, leading to a more alkaline pH that drastically decreases the extent of absorption of minerals and nutrients from the foods we eat —

further creating a negative ecosystem of gut health. A recent study from 2019 stated that the effects of glyphosate not only harmed the gut's microbiome, but it also resulted in some negative effects on the brain, causing imbalances emotionally, neurologically, and promoting progression of neuromuscular disorders.

- **Bisphenol A (BPA):** This compound is well known for its industrial use in creating certain plastics and resins. BPA is typically found in polycarbonate plastics and epoxy resins. We find BPA in a wide array of different food containers in stores, including water bottles. Studies have shown that BPA decreases your intestinal permeability, which allows pathogens and toxins to enter the gut and contribute to Leaky Gut Syndrome. It also attacks the microbiome present in the gut, resulting in alterations in your metabolism. This leads to an imbalance that acts as a precursor to inflammatory conditions of the body like inflammatory bowel disease. BPA also reduces the effectiveness of common chemotherapeutic agents (vinblastine and cisplatin), resulting in the continued multiplication of human breast cancer cells.

Heavy Metals

Heavy metals are another source of toxic potential to the human body. Most of the time, we don't think of the impact we have on our bodies when we get simple procedures like a filling at the dentist. The main toxic effect of heavy metals includes the disruption of the physiological processes associated with gut microflora. Oral lead exposure increases the amount of *E.coli* bacteria present in the gut, which leads to an increased risk of developing illnesses and exacerbating current chronic conditions.

- **Cinnabar is another heavy metal that influences the energy and amino acid metabolic processes**, causing small and irreversible injury to the liver and the kidney. Indirectly, the presence of cinnabar may cause a process that we call oxidative stress (an imbalance between the healthy antioxidants in our body and that of the free radicals that damage our body) to become exacerbated.
- **Mercury, copper, silver-copper alloy, and fluoride** affect antibacterial activity, which is not seen as a positive effect on the gut. This is because destruction of the microbiome and good bacteria present in the gut can cause imbalance and

digestive issues. With exposure to these heavy metals it may allow for some potential pathogens to infiltrate your body. Due to an already weakened immune system, these bacterial species can run rampant throughout the body causing myriad of issues.

Infectious Agents

Molecular mimicry: Infectious agents enter our bodies in a variety of ways and use different mechanisms to do so. One such mechanism is molecular mimicry, which fakes a similarity between foreign parts and those normally present in the human body. One common infectious agent is known as a peptide, and these are particles that make up proteins. Peptides are present in both foreign and human cell structures, giving both types (known as T or B cells) the ability to interact with the immune system cells in the body. This gets into the basics of autoimmunity because we observe how our peptides interact with our cells to mount immune responses against our body's tissue. But what is the possibility of molecular mimicry actually occurring? Is it as common and worrisome as it may seem?

The answer is yes, but only if your gut is unhealthy. Typically, five to six amino acids join to create a peptide, which is necessary should our body initiate an immune reaction.

When we compare all of the known factors involved in creating a peptide, there is only a one in 64 million chance that a peptide forms. In other words, the chances that your body mounts an immune response against your healthy cells is minimalistic at best. But, this is where gut health comes in. An unhealthy gut changes the types of proteins produced in the human body, which heightens the probability of the unusual peptides being generated, which is why an unhealthy gut has increases your chance of developing an autoimmune condition.

Epitope Spreading: Another mechanism is known as "epitope spreading." In order to describe this, we will need to unpack some important concepts. An antigen is a toxic or foreign substance that enters into our body. It is recognized by our body's T-cells, causing our bodies to establish an immune response and release antibodies to fight the antigens.

With those basics in mind, an epitope is the part of the antigen molecule that the antibody attaches itself to, allowing the antibody to defeat and destroy the foreign substance. When epitope spreading occurs, the normal interaction between the antigen and antibody is disrupted. When different epitopes are present, different reactions are produced. A foreign substance may have more than one type of epitope present on its surface, causing different types of immune responses in the body depending on which type of antibodies bind to it. Because an unhealthy gut allows the leakage of substances into the bloodstream, unusual responses are inevitable.

Polyclonal activation: With the next mechanism, polyclonal activation, our bodies have exhausted all of their defenses to ensure that the entire foreign substance is destroyed and removed. Another type of cell in our body, called the B-cell, regulates our natural immune response by adapting to the different types of epitopes presented to the T-cells in our body. B-cells ensure that the antigen is recognized and attacked, accounting for the different epitopes that are present. It achieves this by creating B-cell clones that cover every inch of the foreign substance. This covering allows our bodies to mount an immune response against the foreign substance.

Immune dysregulation: Processes in the body can always go wrong, and this is where immune dysregulation comes in. Sometimes our immune response does not respond in the way that it should, which can be due to genetic or environmental reasons. An example of this is seen with cancers. Instead of an antigen promoting the death and destruction of a foreign body, it facilitates its multiplication and growth, leading to an exaggerated effect that can be linked to the formation of cancer in our body. These types of immune responses are typically unregulated and unre-strained, primarily because the body does not know how to react to it. This is typically seen in severe cases of an unhealthy gut, where your body doesn't recognize it anymore. This causes changes to occur, which have difficulty being understood by your body's regulatory systems.

Stress

Stress is one of the main causes of an unhealthy gut, affecting every part of your digestive system. To our knowledge, the gut is controlled by the central nervous system (CNS) that comprises the brain and the spinal cord. There is another group of neurons that exist in the lining, known as the intrinsic nervous system, which is a subset of the CNS. It is this intrinsic nervous system that is responsible for actions such as swallowing, the release of enzymes to breakdown food, and filtering between nutritious foods and waste. When we find ourselves in stressful situations, our autonomic nervous system (ANS) is activated. The ANS is responsible for monitoring our heartbeat, blood pressure, and breathing rate. It reacts and releases the hormone cortisol that puts our body into a state of high alert. If we experience constant levels of stress, it would result in a constant release of cortisol, leading to a status of awareness that elevates our heartbeat, causes an increase in blood pressure, heightens our breathing, and increases cholesterol levels and muscle tension.

Our digestive system is one of the first systems to be affected when stress activates our "fight-or-flight" response. Our esophagus starts to spasm, we feel nauseous, and there is an increase in acid content in our stomach, followed by diarrhea or constipation. In a stressful instance, blood is directed away from our non-essential organs and to the major organs of the body. This is done to ensure we have enough nutrients and oxygen to remain on high alert. Our stomach is not seen as a major organ by the body, so the decrease in blood flow and oxygen results in cramping, inflammation, and ultimately, an imbalance in the gut bacteria. This will either worsen or increase the likelihood of developing IBS, peptic ulcers, or GERD. This is why it is important to look after your mental health. Keeping yourself calm directly benefits your gut health. Common ways to reduce stress include getting regular exercise, journaling once a week, signing up for a yoga or meditation class, and finding hobbies that you enjoy. This could be painting, taking a walk in nature, or playing with your dogs or cats.

Molds

Molds exist as microorganisms found in the gut, but they can also break and penetrate the intestine's barrier of protection. A subclass of molds known as mycotoxins causes an

LGS that causes widespread inflammation coursing throughout the body. If not treated immediately, this can result in chronic kidney diseases, upset stomachs, diarrhea, and an increased risk of developing cancer.

Medication

Medication plays an important role in the gut health that we experience. The effect that these have is directly related to how long the treatment has been used for. The main manner in which medication affects the health of the gut is through the alteration of the gut's microbiome. The classifications that we will be looking at range from acute use to treatment used for chronic conditions. When we look at proton-pump inhibitors (PPIs), we notice a reduction in the amount of stomach acid that is produced. This completely changes the types of bacteria found within the gut since bacteria have varying growth rates depending on the pH of the environment. Metformin is a form of medication that helps people with type 2 diabetes manage their symptoms. Metformin affects the gut microbiome by decreasing the production of important substances like folate, amino acids, and proteins. Antibiotics, however, fight bacterial infections — which by default result in the destruction of both essential and non-essential bacteria present in the gut. Laxatives trigger mild diarrhea by drawing water into the colon, altering the environment in which bacteria find themselves, resulting in the destruction of some and over-proliferation of others.

Environmental agents

It is important to consider the possibility of how an **environmental agent** could be affecting your gut. If you have tried the elimination diet and are still having issues, why not take a vacation? If your symptoms resolve, then you know that your symptoms are caused by your environment. Here are a few tips on how to foster a gut-friendly environment at home.

Switch to Plant-Based Cleaning Products

Many conventional cleaning products contain a substance called triclosan. Triclosan is an antibacterial and antifungal agent marketed in products such as toothpaste, soaps, and cleaning fluids. However, the Food and Drug Administration (FDA) established that in 2016 all antibacterials that contained triclosan and triclocarban were no longer allowed to be sold to consumers. This was because studies conducted by the FDA showed altered levels of hormone regulation in animals, a contribution to the development of antibiotic-resistant germs, and potential harm to the immune system.

One can only imagine the degree of panic individuals who were using triclosan-containing products were forced into.

Luckily for them, the concentration levels of the triclosan in the products were so low that any side effects that may have been caused were easily reversible. Even so, this anecdote serves as a reminder of the impact substances we take for granted can have on our health.

Avoid Commercial Body Care Products

Body care products contain varying levels of triclosan, phthalates, and parabens, which are absorbed through your skin as they are used. The absorption of these chemicals interferes with gut microbes, resulting in an imbalance. Although these are not present in high enough concentrations to cause serious illnesses, toxins such as parabens can affect thyroid hormone levels, damage your gut health, and expose you to an array of other infectious modalities. I recommend using skincare products that are natural and do not contain microbiome-disrupting chemicals. I also recommend consulting a skincare store to ensure that the products you are purchasing do not include the above compounds.

Eat Organic Produce

Many foods are exposed to pesticides that negatively affect your gut's microbiome. By consuming organic produce, you are lowering the exposure of your body to pesticides and protecting your gut's microbes. One helpful tool is the "Dirty Dozen List". The "Dirty Dozen" lists the 12 foods with the highest amount of pesticide residue before purchasing them. These 12 foods are strawberries, spinach, kale, nectarines, apples, grapes, peaches, cherries, pears, tomatoes, celery, and potatoes. Hot peppers are not on the traditional list but are also known to have high amounts of pesticides.

On the other side of the 'Dirty Dozen' is the 'Clean 15', which includes products with the least amount of pesticide residue before purchase. These 15 foods are avocados, sweet corn, pineapple, onions, papaya, frozen sweet peas, eggplant, asparagus, cauliflower, cantaloupe, broccoli, mushrooms, cabbage, honeydew melon, and kiwi. It is worth mentioning that a small amount of sweet corn and papaya sold may be produced from genetically modified seeds. If you want to avoid these, purchase only organic variants. Organic foods will come at a slightly higher price in supermarkets, but is it worth putting a price on your health?

Reduce Exposure To BPA

By avoiding bottles that are made using BPA and limiting your consumption to canned foods, you can decrease your BPA exposure. Alternatives for water include using a glass or stainless steel water bottle. For food, opting for fresh food instead of canned tastes better and provides a wide array of nutrients and minerals that are essential for promoting good gut health. There are so many toxin-free substances that can be purchased, and you can do a quick search to see which products are available at the stores in your immediate area. Common receipts have traces of BPA in them too. To further decrease exposure, decline a receipt when offered one at stores after your purchases.

Filter Your Drinking and Bathing Water

Tap water is not as pure as many people think. It contains a wide variety of substances, including pharmaceutical drug residue, heavy metals, pesticide residue, and even plasticizers. These amounts vary depending on the effectiveness of your area's environmental filtration systems. In some cases, you could be bathing in water that is contaminated with traces of industrial pollutants and harmful bacteria. I recommend investing in a high-quality water filter that removes these constituents, ensuring that you are feeding your body with nearly pure water. The effects of impure water on our gut are damaging. It can cause diarrhea and other gastric side effects should the substances if ingested frequently and in high amounts.

Tainted water also affects the effectiveness of the supplements that we ingest. If you have a chronic condition and are taking supplements everyday, a drop in efficiency may occur based on the constituents present in tap water. Some supplements do not absorb well when taken with specific minerals, metals, or other substances. Seeing as we don't know the exact composition of every glass of tap water that we drink, it's best to take your supplements with filtered water only.

Consume Prebiotics and Probiotics

Prebiotics and probiotics are essential in aiding the metabolism of toxins in the human body. Prebiotics act as an undigested dietary fiber that feeds bacteria and probiotics, ensuring that the correct amounts of healthy bacteria are present within your gut. Many times, probiotics are given with certain medications such as antibiotics. This helps replenish the healthy bacteria that is destroyed by the antibacterial action of some antibiotics. In studies on prebiotics and probiotics, individuals with inflammatory markers in their bodies are regularly tested over six months to one year. Scientists discovered an immense decrease in the degree of inflammation in those that took prebiotics and probiotics. Those that were responsive to the treatment showed they were getting ill less often, sustained regular bowel habits, and experienced a marked decrease in the extent of side effects from an unhealthy gut.

The next few chapters dive into the details of the most common autoimmune diseases and complications that can arise from an unhealthy gut. We discuss the basics of each disease, the symptoms to watch for, and strategies for preventing and treating each disease. We begin with Leaky Gut Syndrome, a term that is widespread in gut health circles.

5

LEAKY GUT SYNDROME: HOW TO FIGHT BACK AGAINST THE GUT'S #1 ENEMY

Our body's intestinal lining covers 4,000 square feet of surface area — that would cover almost 75% of a football field! When working optimally, some tight barriers and junctions strictly regulate what substances get absorbed into the bloodstream. Unhealthy guts have large cracks or holes that exist within the intestinal lining. This allows partially digested food, toxins, and non-essential bacteria to enter the bloodstream and penetrate the tissues that are present beneath it. The sequence of events that follows includes an inflammatory response that alters the makeup of the gut's microbiome. It is postulated that the modifications in intestinal bacteria and subsequent inflammation may be a strong precursor to the development of several common chronic diseases.

A leaky gut can be associated with a genetic predisposition that results in a person's body becoming more sensitive to changes in the digestive system. Although DNA seems to be the cause of these conditions, it is actually our modern lifestyles that are the main drivers of gut inflammation. When we adopt a western diet that is low in fiber but high in sugar and saturated fats, the leaky gut process is set in motion. If this is combined with stress and the use of alcohol, a leaky gut develops even faster. Many studies show that a leaky gut is associated with a wide array of autoimmune conditions, which we have discussed previously.

When testing to see if you are developing a leaky gut, you may need to follow and document when symptoms occur. Individuals with a leaky gut tend to have gut-specific symptoms like chronic diarrhea, constipation, bloating, and an increase in the amount of gas they produce. They also tend to have nutritional deficiencies because the gut cannot effectively absorb vitamins and minerals from food that is ingested, and this starts a waterfall effect. Due to this lack of nutrients, a poor immune system is established. This makes you more susceptible to contracting infections because your body's defenses are not as strong as they were. Then you start to develop headaches, brain fog, and memory loss, coupled with a sense of excessive fatigue. Skin rashes start to develop and can appear as acne, eczema, or rosacea. You start to crave sugar and carbohydrates because your unhealthy gut contains microbes that need sugar and carbo-hydrates to grow and multiply. Due to the inflammation that is produced, you start developing joint pain, which could lead to arthritis. Your mental health could even be affected by a leaky gut, leading to the symptoms related to depression, anxiety, ADD, and ADHD. Thus, by ensuring that your gut is healthy, the effects of any psychological conditions will be diminished. This is why the saying, "healthy body, healthy mind," rings true.

To understand LGS better, we need to understand the gut barrier. The holding area of the stomach's contents, as well as that of the small intestine, have two completely different systems that contain contrasting compositions. On the one side, you have the digested food that is nutrient-rich, ready to release its vitamins, minerals, and nutrients via the small intestine into the bloodstream. On the other side, you have a sterile bloodstream containing all the essential substances necessary for the optimal functioning of the organs in our body. The challenge is how we efficiently transport nutrients from the nutrient-rich digested food into the bloodstream without allowing the other substances in the stomach and small intestine (acidic juices, viruses, and bacteria) to pass through. The simple answer is to maintain good and constantly monitored gut health habits.

Our gut's barrier consists of two main components. These are *intrinsic* and *extrinsic* barriers. **The intrinsic barrier consists of specific cells that create tight junctions that tie the cells together, ensuring that only molecules that are small enough to pass through the barrier are able to do so.** When looking at the intrinsic barrier, we notice that small toxins and microorganisms, that can traverse this layer of cells, have direct access to the body's bloodstream and access to all major organ systems. Luckily for us, our body planned for this and made a plasma membrane that consists of gut-specific cells called parietal and chief cells. These cells ensure that no acidic components traverse the cell layer and alter the environment in which blood constituents find themselves.

The extrinsic barrier is responsible for the secretions present within the gut. These secretions, like mucus and bicarbonate, are what help maintain this barrier function. The intrinsic gut is reinforced by coating the entire gut with a layer of mucus. Within mucus, there are molecules called mucin that ensure bacteria do not group together, aiding in their removal from the body. The cells present in the gut also secrete bicarbonate that aids in maintaining a neutral pH amongst the cells.

STRATEGIES FOR FIGHTING, REPAIRING, AND DEFEATING LGS

Take zinc

So what can you do to feel better when suffering from LGS? Zinc is an element that plays a necessary role in many of the body's metabolic processes. It's a common ingredient in immune boosters due to its strong effect on our immune systems. Studies performed showed that zinc could strengthen the gut's lining by modifying the tight junctions that ensure adequate permeability is obtained.

L-Glutamine

L-Glutamine is an amino acid that is well known as a reparative substance to the intestinal lining. Studies regarding the use of glutamine in patients with LGS showed great promise and resulted in improved growth and survival rates of intestinal cells while aiding in the regulation of the intestines barrier during periods of high stress. For those of you who enjoy performing high-intensity strenuous exercise, you will be happy to know that a recent study showed that a low dose of oral glutamine right after exercise could reinforce and improve intestinal permeability.

Take probiotics

At this point you are aware of the positive effects of probiotics, but to stress that point even more, a 14-week trial showed that there were much lower levels of zonulin (a marker of gut leakage) present in patients who were on probiotic supplementation than those that were not. Considering LGS is directly related to an unhealthy gut caused by too much bad bacteria, this makes sense. We need to rid the bad bacteria and replace it with the good. It really is as simple as that.

Take scientifically-backed supplements

Fiber and butyrate are important components of a healthy diet. Fiber works similarly to probiotics since it improves the status of the microbiome. When fiber becomes fermented, it creates butyrate, a short-chain fatty acid that stimulates the production of mucus within the gut, as well as improving the strength of the cellular tight junctions of the intrinsic barrier. Deglycyrrhizinated licorice (DGL) studies that have been conducted show promising results and reveal that DGL is a potent anti-inflammatory agent that also enhances mucus production. Curcumin is a plant-based substance that provides spices (like that of turmeric) with its yellow color. Although curcumin isn't absorbed as readily by the body, the small amount that is absorbed shows potent anti-inflammatory effects, providing an explicit benefit towards the functional lining of the gut. Berberine is known as being an LGS supplement due to its antioxidant effects as a bioactive plant-based compound. Studies have commended this compound on also having antioxidant, antibacterial, and antiviral properties. Berberine is already known for its use in the treatment of inflammatory bowel disease (IBD). The use of aloe vera, especially in its juice form, is primarily due to its ability to fight inflammation and soothe the gut. Acting as a supporting agent, it reinforces the mucosal secretions, aiding in the healing of the lining, preventing the development or exacerbation of LGS.

From this list of treatment modalities, it is evident that there are many ways to combat LGS and progress towards a healthy gut. All you need to do is to decide to use them, either by yourself or alongside a health professional.

Change your diet: more fiber + less sugar = happier gut

Although a lot of the treatment modalities consist of supplementation, dietary changes can also be used to treat LGS. Increasing your fiber intake should be your first step. Increasing the amount of fiber that you consume will improve the functioning of the gut microbiome. Start by including fruits, vegetables, and whole grains in your diet. Research shows that sugar is directly related to epithelial barrier dysfunction. With that in mind, I advise decreasing your sugar intake to below 37.5 grams per day for men and below 25 grams per day for women. Current research is also starting to link inflammation caused by processed foods and an increase in permeability of the gut. It is best to steer clear or severely moderate your intake of these types of foods: red meat, dairy products, fried foods, and anything else overly processed. Until the leaky gut is resolved and treated, there will be a constant influx of proteins, bacteria, and toxins leaking into the bloodstream. Without treatment, your unhealthy gut is going to maintain a state of chronic inflammation and heighten the chances of disease development.

Diagnosing Leaky Gut Syndrome

LGS is diagnosed by looking for an increase in the permeability potential of the intestine. You must go to a functional medicine practitioner to perform these tests, and there are three tests that your doctor will likely perform. The first will be an intestinal permeability test using lactulose mannitol. In this test, levels of lactose and mannitol, which are two indigestible sugars, are measured in your urine. The more of these sugars present in your urine, the higher the chance that your intestinal barrier is being broken down.

The second common test is the Immunoglobulin-G (IgG) test. This tests your sensitivity to approximately 90 different foods. This analysis will tell you which foods are most likely food allergies and could be contributing to the diagnosis of a leaky gut. The third test is a zonulin test. The zonulin test focuses on measuring the amount of zonulin antigen present in the body. Because zonulin is directly related to intestinal permeability, having a high amount in the body points toward the intestinal permeability.

Remember to consult a professional

You should always consult a functional medicine practitioner when wanting aid for your gut. Once the tests have been performed, you will need someone qualified to assist you in regulating your diet. This includes recommending the correct type and amount of supplements necessary to ensure the gut's barrier is sealed off and effectively reinforced. LGS can be treated, but it all starts with you deciding to alter your gut health. An unhealthy gut will keep you stuck in a cycle of agony, irritation, and unnecessary expenditure. Make the right choice. Look after your gut and prevent diseases like LGS.

Seeing as LGS is such a common condition and so many people are unaware that they have it, I thought it would be a good idea to give you a week-long dieting plan that is specific for LGS (but can also be used for other gut-related conditions). This is located in the front of the book. Be sure to download it and begin implementing right away.

6

SIBO? WHAT'S THAT?

S mall intestine bacterial overgrowth (SIBO) is a condition in which there is an abnormally large amount of bacteria present within the small intestine. Anatomically, the large intestine should have more bacteria present than the small intestine, primarily due to the other processes (like that of fermentation) that it performs. SIBO is relatively common, so it is important to know the symptoms so you can visit a healthcare practitioner if needed.

Symptoms of SIBO

SIBO contains many of the common symptoms that we associate with gastric conditions. These include bloating, an increase in the production of gas, presence of abdominal pains, cramps, constipation, diarrhea, heartburn, nausea, and even malabsorption. An important distinction of SIBO is what determines whether you have diarrhea or constipation. With SIBO, this is due to what degree of 'unhealthy' your gut displays. The more unhealthy, the more likely you will have diarrhea. While you can treat these symptoms individually, it is important to ensure the underlying condition is treated — else you risk a recurring case of SIBO.

When we discuss malabsorption, it helps to be specific about the vitamins and minerals most affected. SIBO causes steatorrhea, which is known as fatty stools. Fatty stools occur when ingested fats are not adequately broken down and metabolized, combining with your fecal bulk and forming a fatty segment to your excrement. Iron, vitamins B12, D, and K are also affected, and these are important for bone growth, protection against anemia, and blood clotting. For patients that develop osteoporosis (fragile and thin bones), this becomes a cause for concern because bones rely on vitamin D for calcium absorption and the strengthening of weakened bones. This means that osteoporosis patients are more likely to have secondary accidents like hip fractures.

Noticing when SIBO could be causing IBS

People who have IBS may have it as a result of SIBO, but how would you know? When you visit your functional medicine practitioner, they will ask you a few questions to ascertain whether SIBO is the likely cause of the IBS. Aspects that lean toward your IBS being due to SIBO include the following:

- Someone who had an infection that resulted in very serious bouts of diarrhea and stomach cramps likely developed IBS due to SIBO. This is because characteristically SIBO's bacterial overgrowth effect stimulates diarrhea at a much slower rate than IBS. This is why it is important to ensure that the timing of the diarrhea is noted.

- When a patient uses an antibiotic and says that their gut symptoms have improved, we expect this to be due to SIBO. An antibiotic works via its antibacterial action, decreasing the ability of bacterial overgrowth in the small intestine. IBS does not have a direct correlation with bacteria (more specifically, an overgrowth of bad bacteria), which means that antibiotics that have a potent antibacterial effect will directly impact the symptoms present with someone that has IBS via SIBO.

- Because probiotics provide the gut with bacteria, a person with SIBO will most likely have a worsening of their symptoms. This means they will have additional and stronger stomach cramps, more gas production, and severe cases of diarrhea or constipation.

- When someone who has a known diagnosis of celiac disease says that they have not shown an improvement in gut symptoms even when following a gluten-free diet, their chances of SIBO have increased dramatically. This is primarily due to celiac disease being a purely gluten-related form of intolerance, not directly associating with the abundance of bacteria present in SIBO.

- When a person has low iron levels that do not have a likely cause, the patient will probably lean closer to SIBO. This is because SIBO contains bacteria that use the iron for growth and replication purposes. If you are taking iron supplements but still feel the symptoms associated with anemia, you may want to go and get yourself checked for SIBO.

- One of the characteristics of a SIBO gut is a large gas bubble that obscures the pancreas. The bubble exists due to bacteria aiding in the production of gas. As the amount of gas increases, the pressure changes in the gut, causing the gas to accumulate in front of organs like the pancreas that lie behind the gut anatomically.

How SIBO causes IBS symptoms

When we look at the exact manner in which SIBO causes IBS symptoms, two main processes occur. Bacteria can ferment carbohydrates and consume nutrients that are meant to be absorbed by the small intestine, primarily because the overgrowth of SIBO is within the small intestine. This causes malabsorption as the bacteria get in the way of nutrients, minerals, and vitamins' ability to cross the small intestine and enter the bloodstream. During the bacterial fermentation process, two gasses are produced, hydrogen and hydrogen sulfide. These gases cause the symptoms of bloating, pain, and increased gas. Depending on the severity of SIBO, the quantity of gas generated may increase significantly — even to the point of feeling constant bloated when you aren't eating.

SIBO's side effects have a potential impact too, especially in cases where lactose-intolerant people have similar symptoms when they drink lactose-containing products. Pain in the gut is due to the buildup of pressure in the small intestine caused by the fermentation process. Diarrhea or constipation is due to the amount of hydrogen or hydrogen sulfide that is produced. This is associated with heightened amounts of hydrogen production, while some bacteria that produce methane have a unique association with constipation. This can, however, cause large amounts of confusion and complications as if you have bacteria in SIBO that produces both hydrogen and methane. You will start having a mixed response that alternates between diarrhea and constipation. It is this pressure that is created that also aids in GERD as the pressure pushes up the gut, affecting the stomach contents and the esophagus. The manner in which SIBO causes anemia is by the bacteria using the iron as a food source, leading to low amounts available in the bloodstream.

The 3 main types of SIBO-causing bacteria

Three main types of bacteria are common contributors to SIBO. These include *Clostridium*, *E.coli*, and some *Streptococcus* species. How these types of bacteria are tested are different. *Clostridium* is tested with a stool sample, and *E.coli* and *Streptococcus* species need to be cultured in the lab once sterile swabs are taken. This is different from how you diagnose SIBO. To diagnose SIBO, a lactulose breath test is performed. This test works by drinking a sugar lactulose solution. You are then required to breathe into a balloon every 15 minutes for 3 hours. Every time this is done, a sample of the breath in the balloon is tested for the presence of hydrogen or methane gas. This is an accurate way of diagnosing someone with SIBO, especially if their symptom profile fits the clinical outline of SIBO. A simultaneous test is usually performed to see if you have a bacteria called *H.pylori* present in your gut. This bacteria is well known for causing gut disturbances, which include ulcers and gut-based symptoms. If an *H.pylori* infection remains untreated, the ulcers could rupture or the person could have an increased risk of developing gut-based cancer. Ulcer rupture is a medical emergency and requires urgent and immediate attention should it occur.

Treatment options for SIBO

Herbal antimicrobials are seen as good treatment options for people who have SIBO. Examples of these are widely available; they will help curb your symptoms and aid in the resolution of SIBO. Candibactin is a thyme and oregano essential oil that consists of sage and lemon balm extracts. Its main ingredient is thyme oil, which is known to have strong antibacterial properties — especially in cases where there are multiple drug-resistant strains of bacteria present. Dysbiocide is another example of antimicrobial treatment for SIBO. It contains wormwood, yarrow, and dill seed, which are known to exhibit strong antimicrobial activity when used together. Biocide on its own is a herbal supplement that includes bilberry extract along with milk thistle, echinacea, goldenseal, shiitake, lavender oil, and tea tree oil, amongst other components. Many people with SIBO prefer to use their own combinations of herbs. Typically they use either allicin, berberine, oregano, or cinnamon. Atrantil is an over-the-counter supplement with a unique blend of *M.balsamea* (known as peppermint) wild extracts, quebracho, and conker tree. It targets the methane-producing SIBO that are not killed by antibacterial substances.

Reduce fermented foods if you suspect you have SIBO

You should restrict the intake of highly fermentable foods if you suspect you have SIBO. There is an array of SIBO diet maps available, but we are going to provide you with some SIBO-friendly recipes to ensure your symptoms are minimized and your gut begins to return to its normal health. Anyone with SIBO should make an active effort to use some of the recipes listed below while working alongside a functional medicine doctor. Some of the recipes for a SIBO diet can be rather expensive, and this is why it is necessary to have the input of a functional medicine doctor. They can tailor your path to good gut health based on your unique needs and make it as cost-effective as possible.

7

IBS CAUSED BY STRESS

I rritable bowel syndrome (IBS) is a disorder of the large intestine. You may have noticed that the location of the condition allows us to categorize symptoms and facilitate your diagnosis. Signs and symptoms that are related to IBS include cramps around the area of your belly button, an increase in the production of gas present, and either single bouts of or alternating cases of diarrhea and constipation. IBS is a chronic condition and requires long-term management for its symptoms to be alleviated and for your gut to return to a healthy state. Managing your symptoms requires a combination of diet modifications, lifestyle alterations, and stress management.

So when should you see a functional medicine doctor? It is a good idea to visit your healthcare practitioner when you show a constant change in your bowel habits with symptoms of IBS. The symptoms linked to IBS are also related to colon cancer, so stay on the safe side and always get it checked out. Weight loss, diarrhea at arbitrary times at night, bleeding from your rectum, iron deficiency anemia, unexplained vomiting, and difficulty swallowing are all signs that you should make an appointment with your doctor.

The precise cause of IBS is not well known, however, there are factors that contribute to the symptoms of IBS. These start with the muscle contractions in the intestine. The intestine walls are lined with muscles to ensure that the food we eat, the liquids that we drink, and the medication we ingest are moved effectively along the gut to areas of absorption and removal of waste products. These muscles are lined with little hairs that we refer to as 'villi.' The function of villi is to facilitate the movement of substances through your gut and to aid in the removal of residue particles that need to be eliminated.

In IBS, the contractions of these muscles are stronger and can last longer than normal. These longer contractions cause gas, bloating, and diarrhea in people who have IBS. Weak contractions of the intestinal muscles slow the movement of gut contents, leading to hard and dry stools. The nerves that are present in your gut contribute heavily to the discomfort you feel when you have IBS. When your gut stretches due to the presence of gas or stools, your brain sends a signal to overreact to changes that are not the normal occurrence in your gut, resulting in pain when experiencing diarrhea and constipation. Inflammation in the intestines is a marked effect that is directly related to an unhealthy gut. There is an increase in the number of immune-system cells in the intestines, which directly contributes to pain.

This disorder can also develop after a very severe case of diarrhea that may have been caused by another bacteria or virus. With this newfound surplus of bacteria in the intestines, patients may develop SIBO from IBS. Changes in the gut's 'good' bacteria result in an imbalance in the health of the gut. Researchers have been trying to see if there is any basis for the predisposition of IBS and found that individuals who develop IBS have different bacterial compositions in their gut than the general public. The altered composition of bacteria could be due to various reasons, including different genes, environments, and staple foods.

IBS Triggers

IBS also has specific triggers that set off a cascade of symptoms that one would typically experience after being diagnosed with IBS. These include food, hormones, and stress. The role of food, specifically an allergy or intolerance, needs to be distinguished from an individual with IBS. People who experience a worsening of symptoms may suffer even more when eating allergen-containing products including wheat, dairy, citrus fruits, cabbage, milk, and other carbonated beverages.

When considering hormones, women are twice as likely to develop IBS due to the number of hormones that are constantly fluctuating. Women also see their signs and symptoms of IBS worsen, especially right before and during their menstrual cycles. Stress is the most common and worst trigger of IBS, though. When people experience a heightened period of stress, their symptoms become aggravated. However, it is important to mention that IBS is not solely due to stress; it is stress coupled with an array of other factors directly related to the health of your gut. How stress triggers IBS is through the interaction of cortisol and the degree of inflammation that is caused within the gut. Individuals who suffer from chronic stress will notice that their bowel movements are never regular or 'normal.'

Even if your diet is perfect, stress can trigger your IBS symptoms. Irritable bowels have been linked to irritable brains. Studies have shown that there is a direct link to stress and the sensitivity impact of your intestine, the movement of substances through your gut, the secretion of different essential substances, and the permeability of the barriers within your gut. With stress-causing reactions that put you into a high-strung emotional whirlwind, IBS symptoms tend to flare up and are exacerbated by the responses sent from your brain to the gut. Some individuals are put on antidepressants to monitor their stress levels, whether it be emotional or environmental stress. The point is, stress is harmful and will impact your gut negatively. This is why the most integral part of treating someone who has IBS is using a multidisciplinary team of healthcare professionals to ensure they have the best outcomes possible. For example, a patient could use a psychologist for stress and a functional medicine doctor for gut health. There is a strong correlation between those with anxiety, depression, and other psychological conditions and their chances of developing IBS. This is why a functional medicine doctor should inquire about your mental health before making a diagnosis.

Many doctors will ask the question, "What came first, the IBS, or the anxiety?" With stress and anxiety being our body's responses to danger, whether impending or immediate, IBS is directly affected. Remember that there is no cure for IBS, but there *are* definitive ways to decrease its effects and how you react to those effects. Biologically speaking, stress impacts the intestine's internal environment. It decreases the amount of blood that flows to the intestine, increases its permeability, and activates your immune system to call in inflammatory cells that aggregate in the gut — causing IBS symptoms.

Strategies for reducing stress and anxiety

When we look at the connection between stress and IBS, some people will know the source of their stress immediately. Others will take longer to isolate the root of their stress. For those of you dealing with stress, whether you have IBS or not, I advise keeping a journal. In this journal, take note of your daily patterns, including the symptoms that you feel after, during, and before stressful situations. This will help you understand your stress triggers and how well specific interventions work when implemented. Not everyone will be able to identify their stressors by simply doing some introspection — many require cognitive brain therapy, which is performed by a psychologist to get to the root of their stress. Once identified, you can start to take active steps to teach yourself to cope with the stress that specific situations create. Here are some other ideas that when implemented to help deal with your anxiety, especially for those that have IBS:

- **Stress-relieving practices such as meditation or yoga** teach you deep-breathing techniques, forcing you to focus on your thoughts and enabling you to come to terms with your ability to handle stressful environments effectively. The more that we are able to deal with our thought processes, the easier it is to deal with new problems when they arise.

- **Sleep is very important, although most of us don't get enough of it.** Sleeping at least seven to eight hours a night is important to ensure that you have enough energy to get through the day without needing an afternoon nap. When you go to sleep, avoid using electronic devices in bed and keep your bedroom cool and dark. Habits like these will increase your quality of sleep. With today's technology, finding a sleep-tracking application on your phone or smartwatch can give you some insight regarding your sleeping patterns. The importance of regular sleep patterns can also be emphasized using the circadian rhythm. The circadian rhythm is a cycle that regulates the level of sleep we are in as our bodies sleep through the night. There is a misconception that taking a two-hour nap counts toward total sleep. This is incorrect. The total sleep that you obtain is actually classified by the amount of time you spend in a deep or REM sleep.

- **Professional help from a psychiatrist may be needed.** Some people find it difficult to talk to a psychiatrist about their IBS problems, but you should if other techniques don't provide relief. A good psychiatrist can help you manage your stress effectively.

- **IBS support groups** may be of some benefit to those that benefit from community and accountability. IBS is a global problem, connecting with people who are struggling with similar symptoms and hearing how they overcame them can be a huge benefit.

- **Complementary medicine techniques** that focus on pressure points like acupuncture, massage, or reiki have shown to relieve stress in some people, helping them manage their IBS with reduced symptoms.

Set aside some time each day to do something you enjoy. You will be surprised at how much this helps. As a functional medicine doctor, I have patients that meditate, journal, and practice deep breathing exercises to help reduce stress levels. Planning these activities and putting them into your calendar is a way to ensure that you do not forget to do them.

Here are a few hobbies you can explore. These may provide you with renewed satisfaction while decreasing stress. Many have recommended that listening to your favorite music genre for at least half an hour a day can decrease your blood pressure, slow down your heart rate, and calm anxiety and stress. This was researched extensively by Harvard Health, where they even looked at the effect of music on helping heart attack survivors worry less about their health and decreasing the pain in people undergoing surgery. This is why in most dental practices, they give you the option of laying in the chair with headphones on (the added benefit is that you don't hear the noise of the drill). Dancing is also a great stress reliever since our bodies respond to cardio exercise by releasing endorphins (also known as our happy hormones), which gives you a great sense of accomplishment after your session.

Dancing decreases stress by activating the brain's pleasure circuits, whereas music's rhythm helps the person create a bond with the music, alleviating stress in the process. Many individuals have a want for repetition, which is why knitting is seen as a very good stress-reliever. The rhythmic and repetitive motion of pulling yarn or string releases serotonin, which aids in keeping us calm and happy. The amount of focus required distracts you from worrying about your problems, which decreases your blood pressure, slows down your pulse, and helps prevent stress-related illnesses.

Taking a stroll outside allows you to become one with nature, giving you a sense of feeling 'grounded.' It is seen as a positive distraction that ensures that you are not dwelling on a specific problem.

Watching a good movie, or even better, a funny movie ensures that you are focusing on something that isn't your problem.

8

CELIAC = GLUTEN ISSUES

C eliac disease is an immune reaction to eating gluten, a protein commonly found in wheat, barley, and rye. Sometimes called celiac sprue or gluten-intolerance, the immune response that is triggered when someone eats gluten occurs in your small intestine. When we analyze this condition over time, constant gluten ingestion causes a large amount of damage happens to the gut lining. As soon as there is something wrong with the lining of your small intestine (remember your small intestine is the main area for nutrient absorption), the food's minerals and vitamins never get absorbed. When your body doesn't have access to these essential nutrients, it responds to this imbalance with the signs and symptoms associated with celiac disease. These include diarrhea, immense fatigue, weight loss, bloating, and

anemia. If your gut is not taken care of during your diagnosis, severe complications could occur — especially with children, where growth and development can be significantly impaired.

Symptoms and Risks of Celiac Disease

There is no cure for celiac disease, however, for most people following a strict gluten-free diet seems to manage their symptoms and promote intestinal healing. The signs and symptoms that a person with celiac disease experiences are the typical, gut-centric signs and symptoms. However, what many people don't know about celiac disease is that many patients experience seemingly unrelated symptoms. Anemia is a common sign primarily due to the decrease in the amount of iron absorbed in the body, leading to a deficiency. Some patients show a decreased bone density (osteoporosis) or softening of the bone (osteomalacia). These two bone conditions usually result in injury from a fall and admission to the hospital, only for the person to find out that their celiac disease was the main cause for developing their bone disorder. An increase in the person's age will mirror the incidence and severity of the bone density disease. Many people have symptoms related to a weakened immune system, such as itchy, blistery skin rashes, headaches, and fatigue. Tingling of the hands and feet (which may or may not be accompanied by numbness) can also appear, with some patients experiencing problems with balance and remembering facts. Joint pain and a decreased functioning of the spleen can also occur.

Celiac disease can increase chances of infertility and the risk of miscarriage as a result of the harbored calcium and vitamin D absorption as well. Because celiac disease causes damage to your small intestine, there may be instances of pain and diarrhea, especially after eating dairy products that contain lactose. You will only be able to eat dairy products after your gut has healed. Individuals with celiac disease who don't take an active role in their gut's restoration process are at a greater risk of developing an array of different types of cancer, ranging from intestinal to small bowel cancers. Seizures also become rather common in patients with celiac disease, primarily due to the effect that not maintaining a gluten-free diet has on the nerves present in the hands, feet, and brain.

What Causes Celiac Disease

The causes of celiac disease seem to be your genetic composition combined with your body's tolerance to gluten. When the body's immune system interacts with gluten in those that have celiac disease, the precise area of damage is the small hairlike projections (called villi) that line your small intestine. To reiterate, the function of these villi includes aiding in the absorption of the minerals, vitamins, and nutrients from the food that you eat. When these structures are damaged, it doesn't matter how much food you eat, you will not be able to absorb the essential components your body needs. Celiac tends to be more common in people who have chronic conditions that exist within their family lineage. A family member with celiac disease will increase the risk of future successive generations developing the condition. Those with Type 1 diabetics, down syndrome, Turner syndrome, thyroid diseases, and Addison's disease also have a greater chance of developing celiac disease. Although it is important to mention that some individuals may have heightened sensitivity due to gluten ingestion, meaning that the symptoms they experience may be worse than those of someone who isn't as sensitive to gluten.

It is said that one in 100 people worldwide will have celiac disease, affecting an estimated three million Americans. In a study that was conducted, 97% of those that had been diagnosed with celiac disease were not aware of their diagnosis. They misread their unhealthy gut as a normal bodily reaction, not seeing the need to seek treatment. Our best defense against Celiac disease is eating gluten-free, and responses to a gluten-free diet vary from person to person. Some people who have celiac disease show immediate relief when they cut gluten out of their diet, while others can struggle for months before obtaining a satisfactory level of relief.

How to Approach Your Diet When Suffering from Celiac Disease

Rye, barley, brewer's yeast, wheat starch, malt, triticale, as well as wheat (this includes Khorasan, semolina, wheat berries, and durum) need to be completely avoided and eliminated from your current diet. You also need to be very careful with what you purchase in the supermarket. You need to ensure that pasta, cereal, bread, desserts (cake and cookies), sauces and soups, have the 'gluten-free label on them. It is important to also take into consideration that gluten isn't only present in foods. You may find traces of gluten in some medication, vitamin supplements, lip balm, communion wafers, eggs, play dough, toothpaste, and even mouthwash.

Gluten-free eating is far from tasteless, though. You can eat meat, fish, fruits and vegetables, beans and lentils, nuts and seeds, rice and potato flour, quinoa, sorghum, tapioca, and much more. I also recommend taking supplements when eating gluten-free. It's easy to overlook nutrients when making such a big change to your diet. Your functional medicine doctor will most likely ensure that you are placed on iron, vitamin D, calcium, and zinc supplements along with a multivitamin that you will need to take daily. And if you're still skeptical about how tasty food can be when eating gluten-free, make sure to download our delicious gluten-free recipes.

9

GERD

What is GERD?

Gastroesophageal reflux disease (GERD) happens when contents from your stomach move up into your esophagus. Many people refer to GERD as acid reflux or acid regurgitation. It is only when reflux occurs more than two times per week that it is suggested to visit your functional medicine doctor and find out if you might have GERD. Research shows that GERD affects one in five Americans, and if left untreated can cause an abundance of serious complications. Patients report that reflux feels like a burning in your chest that can radiate upward to your neck. This feeling is what we refer to as heartburn. Many describe having GERD as re-tasting the food you have already eaten, developing a sour or bitter taste in your mouth, or having a lump in your throat. GERD even has the potential to cause breathing problems like chronic coughs and can exacerbate the symptoms of asthma.

Causes of GERD

The causes of GERD are widely related to the failure of our body's structures, specifically the lower esophageal sphincter (LES), which is the area that connects your esophagus to your stomach. The LES is a band of muscle that relaxes when you swallow, allowing the food you are eating to enter into the stomach. After swallowing, the muscular band tightens and closes up again, ensuring that there is no back-flow of stomach contents during the mixing process (also known as churning). Acid reflux occurs when your LES does not tighten up correctly, resulting in digestive juices and other contents from your stomach to rise back up into your esophagus.

Treating GERD

Your functional medicine doctor will analyze your symptoms, encourage you to make changes to your eating habits, and recommend some lifestyle modifications. They might also suggest herbal remedies and supplements to help you when altering your eating habits. If there is no response to non-invasive treatment, then surgery may be recommended. However, proton pump inhibitors (PPIs) do not eliminate the reflux associated with GERD, as it is more related to the acid component of the stomach's juices. Therefore, the use of PPIs to treat GERD is generally (talk to your doctor) avoided since PPIs simply relieve heartburn, a symptom that can be managed without the use of medication.

When someone has been on a PPI for a long time, they should be weaned off of it as soon as possible (consult with doctor) while treating the underlying causes of GERD.

Here are some therapies that address the causes associated with GERD:

- **You can improve the LES tone** to ensure the contents of the stomach do not backtrack into the esophagus. Try gargling exercises such as a dry gargle or a hard swallow. With a dry gargle, you pull your tongue back during a gargle and hold it for three to four seconds. It's easiest to pretend that you are gargling with mouthwash. You will do a dry gargle approximately 15 to 20 repetitions at a time. With a hard swallow, you are squeezing the muscles when swallowing. Many like to envision themselves swallowing a big chunk of meat or a golf ball. The hard swallow will be performed approximately 10 to 20 repetitions at a time.

- **Focus on improving gastric (the biological term for the stomach) emptying and motility** within your gut to decrease the amount of stomach contents available to move back into the esophagus. As you decrease the contents, you are also reducing the chances of cellular damage occurring in the esophagus.

- **Protection of the lining of the esophagus** is important as the lining is not meant to interact with acidic contents, especially from the stomach's juices with very high acid content.

- **Get rid of ulcers.** Ulcers may be present in the stomach due to the lack of a protective lining. These should be treated immediately to ensure that no further complications occur.

- **Lower PPI intake gradually.** When a PPI is stopped, it should not be halted immediately and the dose should be gradually lowered over time to allow your body to regulate its internal balances effectively. It is highly recommended that instead of using a PPI, you switch to a herbal remedy with proven treatment benefits for GERD. Make sure to consult with a doctor before attempting this.

Diet is an important aspect when we look at gut health and is particularly important when treating GERD. Regionally, the incidence of GERD in Asia is 5% of the population compared to the 10-20% of people in the western world that have GERD. Researchers think this is due to obesity but research is rapidly being done to investigate this further.

GERD is known for causing cells in your esophagus to multiply profusely, ultimately resulting in one cell turning into a different cell type. We refer to this change from one to another as 'metaplasia.' Medically, when this occurs in the esophagus due to GERD, it is called Barrett's esophagus. The importance of obtaining treatment for GERD cannot be emphasized enough because if no treatment is obtained, it will most likely result in the formation of an adenocarcinoma (a form of cancer).

How to Test for GERD

To confirm if you have GERD, a physical exam is performed and a list of symptoms is checked by your doctor. A procedure may take place to confirm the diagnosis and check for GERD complications. A barium swallow is one such test where a patient is required to drink a barium-infused solution, where an x-ray is conducted to obtain imaging of your upper digestive tract. An endoscopy may also be performed, which is when doctors place a flexible tube with a tiny camera on its end inside your esophagus. This tube is used to examine your esophagus and retrieve a piece of tissue for diagnostic purposes. An esophageal manometry test may also be done, which is a test where a flexible tube is used to measure the strength of your esophageal muscles, providing you with a good interpretation of the strength of the LES as well as the chances of GERD being present. The monitoring of pH is also important since stomach acid will drop your pH levels, providing a more concrete diagnosis of GERD.

Many risk factors can predispose one to GERD. Obesity is a solid indicator of potentially developing GERD, which is a cause of concern given the levels of obesity not only in America but around the world. Other risk factors include pregnancy, hiatal hernias, and connective tissue disorders. Lifestyle behaviors can also increase your risk of developing GERD. Smoking and eating multiple large meals can act as precursors to GERD. This, combined with lying down or going to sleep shortly after eating, provides a recipe for GERD development. Eating certain types of food, especially deep-fried spicy foods, will not only negatively affect your gut in other ways but also increase your risk for developing GERD. Regular use of soda, coffee, and alcohol are also associated with GERD. Medications with anti-inflammatory effects such as aspirin and ibuprofen have the potential of causing stomach ulcers, a common complication associated with GERD.

Complications due to GERD won't be serious as long as they are treated, but when left alone they can lead to life-threatening health problems. Esophagitis is a common complication as the constant interaction of the acid environment with your esophageal lining can cause an inflammation cascade and inflame your esophagus. The development of an esophageal stricture can also occur when your esophagus narrows or tightens, making swallowing difficult. Tooth enamel erosion, gum disease, and other dental problems are also common due to the reflux of the acid contents reaching into your mouth.

How to Treat GERD

To decrease your chances of developing complications, treatment is needed. I recommend looking at your diet and seeing what may trigger GERD-related symptoms. Although dietary triggers will vary from one person to the next, many of the common instigators are high-fat foods, spicy foods, chocolate, citrus fruit, pineapple, garlic, mint, onion, alcohol, coffee, tea, and soda. Avoiding these foods will provide a good foundation for the relief of GERD.

Make any necessary lifestyle changes

Your practitioner will suggest these lifestyle changes since they also promote good gut health. If you smoke, your top priority should be to quit. Not only for GERD but also for the array of other health complications. Losing excess weight, eating smaller meals, and avoiding the temptation of lying down after eating ensures optimized digestive processes as well. By avoiding tight clothes, you ensure that no added external pressure is being put on your body's extremities, decreasing the chances of a GERD episode. Using these relaxation techniques as well as avoiding foods and drinks that trigger your symptoms should lower the frequency of GERD episodes.

Try to reduce your anxiety

Anxiety can also make your GERD symptoms worse. Limiting your exposure to experiences (whether these are comfortable or uncomfortable), people, and places that make you feel anxious will help you lower your anxiety. By watching a few YouTube videos or asking a medical professional, you can discover relaxation techniques like meditation or deep breathing that can also provide relief. Anxiety can also be reduced by healthily adjusting your sleeping habits, implementing an exercise routine, and adding in other positive lifestyle behaviors that distract you from anxious thoughts. If you suspect you may have an anxiety disorder, you can seek treatment like group therapy, medication, or a combination of the two.

Understanding pregnancy and its relationship to GERD

Pregnancy can increase your chances of experiencing an acid reflux episode. If you were diagnosed with GERD before you became pregnant, it is important to know that your symptoms may worsen. The hormonal changes that occur during pregnancy have a direct effect on the muscles of your esophagus. The muscles of your esophagus will relax more frequently, creating a more consistent pathway for your stomach acid to reflux into your throat. With the presence of a growing fetus, the pressure is also placed over the stomach area, further increasing the risk of stomach acid entering into your esophagus. Some medications that are used to treat acid reflux may not be safe during pregnancy. By consulting with your healthcare professionals, you will be able to identify the best course of treatment.

Understanding asthma and its relationship to GERD

Research has reported that more than 75% of people with asthma also experience GERD. The research is ongoing in order to understand the exact relationship between the two, but GERD may worsen the symptoms of asthma. It has also been published that

GERD-related symptoms are more common in individuals who have IBS than the general population. In many individuals, drinking alcoholic beverages acts as a direct trigger to making the GERD symptoms experienced worse. Depending on the extent of your GERD symptoms, the effect that minimalistic alcohol consumption has on your body will be different from person to person. Even if you combine alcohol with mixers, there is a high chance that the mixers themselves will also exacerbate your GERD symptoms.

Consider using supplements

Using supplements may alleviate GERD symptoms as well help people remove their dependency on acid-blockers. Deglycyrrhizinated licorice (DGL) is a remedy used for GERD, ulcers, and inflammation of the gut. This specific supplement provides an anti-inflammatory effect without having any negative effects on the electrolyte balance in the body. This imbalance is common when using normal licorice. The main factor that influences the effectiveness of DGL is the time of the day that it is taken. Studies show that the best time to take DGL is to chew it six to eight times per day, at least 30 minutes before or two hours after a meal. Other supplements consist of plantain and apple pectin, mucilaginous substances that aid in soothing the esophageal mucosa. Cinnamon is also a major ingredient and is well known for its antibacterial properties. Supplements that contain green tea extract and astaxanthin provide a dual antioxidant and anti-inflammatory benefit. Arabinogalactans are added to supplements to stimulate the immune system as a prebiotic, ensuring that helpful bacteria are synthesized. This works with D-mannose to suppress the mucosal adhesion of harmful bacteria present in the gut.

Melatonin is a supplement that is best known for its effect as a sleep and circadian rhythm regulator. Although effective in controlling sleep, melatonin has also shown promise when administered for GERD. Melatonin can suppress excess acid production in the gut, establish a protective layer, and ensure there is no destruction caused by stress. Studies suggest that taking three to six milligrams of melatonin at bedtime will significantly decrease your GERD symptoms.

Iberogast is a German formulation that was initially used for indigestion. It uses a concoction of herbs including iberis amara, angelica, chamomile, caraway fruit, St. Mary's thistle, balm leaves, peppermint leaves, celandine, and licorice root. When all of these herbs act together, they result in a potent anti-inflammatory effect that coexists with an antispasmodic, antibacterial, and pro-motility effect. This gives evidence to the use of iberogast in GERD symptom relief. This liquid formulation also promotes gastric emptying and intestinal transit, making your gut's food transition process smoother. Due to the antibacterial action of Iberogast's components, it has also been shown to aid in the alleviation of symptoms associated with SIBO. Users should take note that Iberogast contains peppermint and should only be used by those who are sure it isn't a trigger for their GERD symptoms. Iberogast should only be taken under the supervision of a doctor. Do not try this supplement randomly.

While we most often associate aloe with burn treatments, it's also well-known as a gut healer. When looking for an aloe product, it is important to limit additives like sugar and other flavoring agents that could irritate the gut instead of aiding in the alleviation of GERD symptoms. Probiotics have not had an official study performed to see how it directly impacts GERD. However, from what we know about probiotics, its ability to balance out the bacterial ecosystem in the gut is most likely beneficial, even though it may not alleviate GERD symptoms directly.

The final words on GERD

GERD has received a lot attention lately. It's a debilitating condition, but the seriousness of GERD decreases once you know the correct treatment modalities. GERD makes people very uncomfortable, but if you follow the above treatment and steps to consolidate and prevent GERD, you will have nothing to fear.

This disorder has the potential to be associated with a wide variety of other gut conditions, including the different ones we discussed above. Don't waste anytime in resolving GERD. The longer you let it affect you, the more drastic the consequences become.

DOES THE BRAIN CONTROL THE GUT OR VICE VERSA?

Now that we have covered many of the major diseases that can arise from an unhealthy gut, let's talk about the brain and its relationship to the gut. The brain provides stimulation to different nerves around our body, including the gut. With this in mind, we can establish a causal link between psychological disorders and their effects on the abdomen (causing stomach problems to arise). This provides truth to the sayings, "This makes me feel nauseous" and "I feel like I have butterflies in my stomach." The gut is very sensitive to our emotions; whether it be anger, sadness, anxiety, or happiness, our gut will react accordingly.

The brain has a direct link to the stomach and the intestines. An example of this is when our stomach produces juices to digest our food before we have physically eaten anything.

This occurs in response to our thought processes in the brain, stimulating our gut to prepare for food, although it is worth mentioning that the intestine provides feedback to the brain as well. When a person finds themselves in a state of intestinal distress, it could be due to their anxiety, stress, or relapse into depression. This becomes relevant when a person experiences an upset stomach but has no apparent reason why (i.e., a physical cause such as expired food being ingested cannot be found). This ultimately shows that a bidirectional pattern is established between the brain and gut function, where signals here can influence the brain and vice versa.

When we are stressed, the immune system finds it more difficult to fight against foreign organisms that enter into our bodies. In this way, we become more prone to developing infections due to this weakened defense mechanism. This is all related to the hormone cortisol that is secreted by our body when we are in a stressful environment or mindset. Cortisol serves a variety of different functions in our body. These functions include the regulation of blood sugar levels, regulating our metabolism, as well as reducing inflammation present in the body. However, cortisol also weakens our immune system, decreasing the number of cells that fight infection. So, when we are stressed, we become more susceptible to infections that we would have been able to fight off if we were in a non-stressed state. We are also more susceptible to coping mechanisms when stressed. These coping mechanisms include smoking and drinking, which are very unhealthy substances for your gut.

FOODS THAT CONTRIBUTE TO BRAIN INFLAMMATION AND OTHER DETRIMENTAL EFFECTS

Fast food

Along with this, certain food types will result in a detrimental effect on your immune system which in turn causes brain inflammation. Fast food is one of these exact food types. It results in your body being in a constant state of 'high alert' which biologically causes your cortisol secretion to do the same, decreasing your immune system's defense mechanisms indefinitely. Consistently eating foods that are high in sugars and low in fiber result in there being a new normal established, which contains an increased level of brain inflammation. Instead of eating fast food, use that money to buy a smoothie, snack on some nuts, or if you're really craving it, try homemade organic beef burgers with sweet potato fries.

MSG

Foods that contain MSG can cause rather harsh effects on your brain and nervous system. It does this by causing imbalances in your hypothalamic pituitary adrenal (HPA) axis, which are essential organs in the nervous system team (where these organs regulate immune cells, hormones and brain function). MSG causes a severe lack of oxygen in these organs, causing them to produce fewer fighter cells. MSG also causes a marked imbalance in your interleukins, which is a substance released by the body as a signal that an infection is present. What is great about cutting MSG out of your diet is that the damage on your HPA axis is reversible if caught early enough — which is partly why your primary focus should always be on your diet and gut health. Many people enjoy the taste of MSG because it gives an 'umami' type of taste. Luckily, this is easily substitutable with natural alternatives that include meat broths, high-quality cheese, mushrooms, and other fermented foods.

Alcohol

Alcoholic beverages, when ingested regularly, reduce the effectiveness of your immune cells, making it easier for you to contract infections. Alcohol also affects your hormone levels, disrupts your circadian rhythm, and further impacts your immune system. A good night of sleep is essential for the optimal functioning of not only the human body but for cognition as well. There is a proportional relationship with the amount of sleep you get and your ability to fend against infections, think clearly, and have good cognitive health.

Instead of reaching for hard liquor, it has been proven that drinking beer and wine in moderation can actually give your immune system a little boost (this with the added effect of it decreasing your chances of having a heart attack). However, going without alcohol is still ideal, and I do not mean this as an endorsement of drinking.

Foods grown with pesticides

Foods that contain pesticides or that are artificially ripened do not give you the full extent of the health properties that some foods provide. Our gut consists of immune cells and have more cells than any other part of the human body. Some say that our gut contains up to 80% of our body's total immune function. In this way, the good bacteria in our gut play an important role in establishing and maintaining the gut barrier, ensuring that undesirable bacteria and environmental toxins do not come into contact with the body's internal environment, especially the brain. I recommend switching from these artificially ripened fruits and vegetables to strictly organic. The difference between artificially ripened foods and those that let nature take its course is the amount of prebiotic fiber present. When we eat foods that have naturally ripened, the amount of lectin (the substance that promotes color change in fruits and vegetables) decreases, minimizing the chance of our microbial balance in the gut being disrupted. Plants that grow out of season are often ladened with pesticides that harm the gut's micro-biome. This further increases the chances of brain inflammation occurring leading to decreased cognition, brain fog, headaches, anxiety, and depression. Instead of purchasing food because it looks good, make sure that your fridge is stocked with organic foods in season. Try shopping at your local farmer's market to start.

Caffeine

Caffeine is a staple for many in the mornings. While it may seem to make the early hours easier, it can have some unwanted effects on your brain. The boost of energy it gives you in the morning results in an increase in cortisol levels, lowering your threshold to infections since you constantly have a high level of cortisol flowing through your body. Instead of drinking coffee all day, have your coffee cup in the morning but then substitute your subsequent cups of coffee with beverages that have a less caffeine, like tea. Caffeine has also shown to be affiliated with high levels of diarrhea due to the stimulant effect that it provides our body with. When we use stimulants, our gut's normal functional patterns become disrupted, further establishing a negative impact. The key to caffeine intake is moderation. I suggest to all my patient to cycle off of caffeine every four weeks to ensure optimal function.

When it comes to brain and cognitive function, the message that we are given is crisp and clear. If we take good care of our brain, it will take good care of us. The first step is to avoid or limit the foods we have just discussed. I advocate shopping smart. Purchasing the most expensive products to enhance your brain does not mean your brain will be boosted more than someone who bought fresh produce from their local supermarket. When making dietary options that benefit our brains, we need to think smart and long term.

Maintaining your gut microbiome is one of the most important ways to maintain your health with the aided use of prebiotics, probiotics, and gut-healthy habits. Prebiotic-rich foods create a welcoming environment for beneficial bacteria in the gut. It nourishes the bacteria and helps it thrive. It is, therefore, of utmost importance that prebiotic foods are constantly added to your meals. Examples of these foods include dandelion greens, banana, onions, and garlic. These dietary changes, coupled with ways to reduce stress, increasing exercise capabilities, and getting plenty of rest, will result in optimal gut health.

Cognitive and emotional dysfunctions place an increased burden on our society. The exact factors and underlying mechanisms that precipitate these disorders are not entirely understood. It is known that brain dysfunction typically presents with a metabolic disorder (e.g., obesity) and poor dietary habits. This means that the degree at which brain dysfunction occurs will correlate to our dietary habits. So, the healthier and cleaner diet you have, the more optimal your brain function will be.

Western Diets negatively affect the brain and body

When we look at adults in developed countries, it is well known that they are consuming diets that are much higher in saturated fats and refined sugars. This is what we commonly see in the western diet. Recent reports have shown that approximately 12% of American adults' daily intake comes from saturated fats, with 13% from added sugar. These values exceed the recommended amount of 5-10%, which I believe is still too high, that has been stipulated by the US Department of Agriculture, as well as the Department of Health and Human Services. We can expect that there would be a much larger incidence of obesity and brain dysfunction as a result of these dietary habits. This diet has also coincided with alarming rates of Parkinson's and Alzheimers, and the number of obese people has only risen. 37% of the US population is obese, a marked increase of the 13% seen in the 1960s.

These statistics are alarming because associated conditions such as Parkinson's, Alzheimer's, dementia, cardiovascular disease, metabolic syndrome, and type 2 diabetes are all rising. With the amount of inflammation that is caused by food in the western diet, there is now an explicit association between obesity and mild cognitive impairments (including dementia). Short-term consumption (approximately one to seven days) of an unhealthy diet triggers inflammatory processes in the brain, and it can affect the center that controls the hormone release in our bodies known as the hypothalamus. With the amount of information we have about obtaining long and short-chain fatty acids from your diet, these saturated fatty acids have been shown to pass into the hypothalamus and cause an inflammatory response. Although, what can be confusing is that when the region of the brain that is focused on memory and learning, the hippocampus, was not affected, the effects that this segment of the brain has on our body's functioning becomes impaired. As discussed previously, the HPA axis plays a major role in a wide array of bodily functions. Inflammation of the hypothalamus ultimately leads to symptoms associated with poor cognition, anxiety, depression, brain fog, increased weight gain, and autoimmune diseases.

The point is, what you eat will affect your memory as well as your mood. Fluctuations in blood sugar levels can cause many memory problems, including brain fog, headaches, and blurry vision. With the current research on the effect of sugars on cognitive function, Alzheimer's disease is starting to be called type 3 diabetes. With cognitive function being based on the abundance of vitamins and minerals present, it is imperative to have proper absorption to have a stable mood. This will enable you to not only understand your behavioral issues but also give you the confidence to lead a healthy and active lifestyle.

Further research in this field has led to studies of how the human gut microbiome impacts human brain health. Some of the manners in which the human brain is impacted are as follows:

- **Structural components of bacteria, such as lipopolysaccharides, provide low-grade stimulation of our body's innate immune system.** Excessive stimulation due to the presence of a bacterial dysbiosis, small intestinal bacterial overgrowth, or increased intestinal permeability may produce systemic or central nervous system inflammation. When we are in a constant state of inflammation, the chance for bowel diseases to develop is likely.

- **Bacterial proteins may cross the blood brain barrier with the antigens that our body produces.** This leads to stimulating a dysfunctional response where the adaptive immune system attacks the brain. These dysfunctional responses have a marked impact on our brain's ability to function effectively and with minimal side-effects. If these abnormal responses are not rectified, we begin to develop constitutional symptoms that fit the illness profile, including brain fog, feeling lethargic, memory problems, depression, and anxiety.

- **Bacterial enzymes may produce neurotoxic metabolites, which include the likes of D-lactic acid and ammonia.** The metabolites that we believe are beneficial have the potential to cause neurotoxicity. An example of such a metabolite is short-chain fatty acids. Neurotoxins are substances that alter the function of the nervous system. This altering damages brain cells or the nerves which carry signals around the body. When neurotoxicity is not rectified, along with the constant exposure to a neurotoxic substance, the prevalence of some disorders may increase. Examples of these disorders include impaired intelligence, impaired regulation of emotional responses, behavioral problems including attention deficit and hyperactivity disorders, depression, anxiety, memory formation, impaired physical coordination, and increased risk of neurodegenerative disorders such as Parkinson's and Alzheimer's diseases.

- **Gut microbes can produce hormones and neurotransmitters that are identical to those produced by humans.** Bacterial receptors for these hormones influence microbial growth and virulence. The alteration in the levels of hormones that are produced presents a large difficulty to the homeostatic mechanisms of our body. Our gut microbes synthesize and secrete a number of hormones, including Cholecystokinin (CCK), Peptide YY (PYY), Glucagon-like Peptide-1 (GLP-1), Gastric Inhibitory Polypeptide (GIP), and 5-Hydroxytryptamine (5-HT). The function of these hormones is regulatory in nature, meaning that they have key regulatory roles in metabolic processes, including insulin sensitivity, glucose tolerance, fat storage, and appetite.

Through these varied mechanisms, gut microbes shape the architecture of sleep and stress reactivity of the hypothalamic-pituitary-adrenal axis. They influence your memory, mood, and cognition. These become clinically relevant when the gut microbes influence the disorder progression and resolution. Examples of these conditions include, but are not limited to, alcoholism, chronic fatigue syndrome, fibromyalgia, and restless legs syndrome. Currently, the role of gut microbes in multiple sclerosis and the neurologic manifestations of celiac disease is still being studied.

The brain plays a pivotal role in the establishment and management of the hypothalamic-pituitary-adrenal (HPA) axis. It is for this reason that more information surrounding it should be shared in order for you to better understand how the brain is linked to our body's processes. The HPA axis is our central stress response system. Whether we are emotionally stressed, physically stressed, or chronically stressed, the HPA axis will always be our body's first mechanism of response. The HPA axis is a representative system that consists of functions that stem from both the central nervous system and the endocrine system.

This system works in a fairly straightforward manner, with logical reactions based on the increase or decrease in the constituents of the HPA axis. It is responsible for the neuroendocrine adaptation component of the stress response. When we experience stress, the typical response is characterized by the hypothalamic release of corticotropin-releasing factor (CRF). Remember, our hypothalamus, along with the pituitary gland in our brain, are responsible for the amount and types of hormones that are produced in our body.

CRF is also known as corticotropin-releasing hormone (CRH), and understanding the mechanism of how CRF works can be rather tricky. I am going to attempt to explain it in the simplest way possible. When CRF binds to the CRF receptors on the anterior pituitary gland, the result is the release of adrenocorticotropic hormone (ACTH). ACTH then binds to receptors on the adrenal cortex and stimulates the adrenal release of cortisol. We are already well-versed on our friend cortisol's effects on the inflammatory processes in the gut, which lead to an increased chance of leaky gut syndrome (LGS) development. In response to stressors, cortisol will be released for several hours after encountering the stressor. How this links to gut health is based on the frequency that the specific stressor presents itself. What usually occurs is that at a certain blood concentration of cortisol, a negative feedback response to the hypothalamus is activated. It is at this point that systemic homeostasis returns.

With repeated exposure to stressors, the human body becomes used to the stressor with repeated and sustained HPA axis activation. The result is unhealthy levels of cortisol that are constantly present for extensive periods. Your body's immune system begins to weaken over longer periods; you become susceptible to a wide array of infections, and you cannot function optimally.

Therefore, it is important to support healthy cortisol levels in order to ensure the hypothalamus and pituitary glands maintain the appropriate level of sensitivity to the negative feedback of cortisol. When we secrete epinephrine and norepinephrine when placed in an 'alarm state,' our adrenal medulla becomes affected. It is the presence of the alarm chemicals in combination with the persisting HPA axis and its secretions of CRF, ACTH, and cortisol that place our body's into high alert.

Interestingly, with aging, the hypothalamus and pituitary are less sensitive to negative feedback from cortisol. Both ACTH and cortisol levels rise as we age, which fits with the clinical pictures that we readily obtain with older people. Older people develop gut problems much faster than younger individuals. In this way, the older generation is more susceptible to infections due to a high level of cortisol that persists as the aging process progresses. There is even a gender aspect to the levels of cortisol that are produced. Older women will secrete more cortisol in response to stress than older men. Researchers are attributing this to the levels of active estrogen that women possess. This also explains why young women produce lower levels of cortisol when confronted with stress in relation to young men.

In conclusion, we can see how the gut-brain axis has a major influence on our overall quality of life. Living with issues such as brain fog, headaches, anxiety, and depression is not a life at all, and I hope you see how gut health is imperative to resolving these issues. To create a life full of clarity and health, you must start with what you feed your body. Treat your gut with the respect it deserves, and it will pay you back with a life of the highest quality.

BASIC FIVE PILLARS OF THE PROCESS TO HEALING YOUR GUT

T hroughout this book, you have been handed an extensive amount of information. Some of it may have required you to read the sentence twice, or maybe even three times to grasp the concept adequately. This chapter is about zooming back out. We're going to cover the *five* pillars that encompass resolving your gut dysfunction. To have an immediate impact on your health, follow these steps in order.

STEP 1: REDUCE INFLAMMATION AND OXIDATION

Increased inflammation negatively affects our gut. Avoiding refined carbohydrates such as white bread or pastries, fried foods, soda and other sweetened beverages, red meat, processed meat, margarine, will decrease inflammation in the gut significantly, ensuring that you are on your way to a healthier gut. Unhealthy foods also contribute to weight gain, which in itself is a strong risk factor for inflammation.

How we combat inflammation is through replacing foods that cause inflammation with the opposite. Examples of healthy foods include fatty fish (salmon, tuna, and sardines), nuts (almonds and walnuts), herbals, olive oil, fruits (strawberries, cherries, and blueberries), and green leafy vegetables (collards, kale, and spinach). These foods are associated with a lower risk of cardiovascular disease and diabetes. We also want to be mindful of the hidden inflammatory ingredients that may be present in some of the foods and meals that we eat.

Supplements may be necessary to decrease the degree of inflammation that our gut experiences. Zinc is a supplement that plays a necessary role in many of the body's metabolic processes. It boosts the immune system and contributes to an anti-inflammatory effect toward the gut while strengthening the lining of the gut. L-Glutamine is an amino acid that acts as a reparative substance to the intestinal lining. It responds to severe cases of stress, increasing the reparative potential of gut cells by decreasing inflammation and ensuring that damage to your gut is effectively taken care of. Fiber and butyrate are important constituents and are essen-

tial components of a healthy diet. Fiber acts by strengthening the gut's microbiome. When fiber is fermented, it
enhances the tight junctions between intestinal cells while
also establishing a layer of mucus as a protective mechanism.
Deglycyrrhizinated licorice (DGL) is a potent anti-inflammatory agent that shows an increase in mucus production.
Some supplements contain all the aforementioned products,
making this process much easier than taking them all individually.

STEP 2: IMPROVE NUTRITIONAL LEVELS

We want our bodies to be in the best shape it can be. When
we feel good, we are more inclined to get work done
throughout the day. With that being said, we want to ensure
that we are eating the correct foods that allow our gut's good
bacteria to flourish. The basic idea is to eat a variety of
different food types. This leads to a diverse microbiome in
your gut. You want to ensure you are eating some high-fiber
foods, which include: raspberries, artichokes, broccoli,
chickpeas, lentils, and whole grains. Studies have shown that
by including enough of these foods in your diet, the growth
of some disease-causing bacteria is prevented. Eating some
fermented foods can definitely strengthen your gut's microbiome, too. Yogurt, kimchi, kombucha, and sauerkraut are
examples of fermented foods that are rich in the bacteria

type known as *Lactobacilli,* which has scientific evidence of benefiting the gut. When you have more *Lactobacilli,* you will have a decrease in *Enterobacteriaceae,* which is a type of bacteria that is known to be associated with inflammation and chronic diseases.

It is important to stay away from artificial sweeteners, as they negatively affect your blood sugar levels. An example is aspartame, which resulted in a decrease in weight gain but increased blood sugar levels and impaired insulin response. For people who have diabetes, this can become a life-threatening situation.

When you focus on including prebiotics, probiotics, polyphenols, and whole grains into your diet, you are bound to make your gut very happy. These all promote gut health directly within the bacterial microbiome, and many have the effect of promoting the good bacteria and preventing the bad. Through establishing a proper nutritional balance in your body, healing of an unhealthy gut will occur.

STEP 3: MINIMIZE STRESS

Minimizing stress requires a multifaceted approach. We start by eliminating foods that result in inflammation in the body. These are specifically foods that are high in saturated fats and refined sugars. Remember, these foods increase the permeability of your intestine, causing bacteria to enter into your bloodstream, resulting in a preventable autoimmune response. Your body can heal when these foods are avoided. Ensuring that you stay away from harmful toxins, including artificial sweeteners, red meat, alcohol, and smoking will decrease the toxic products formed in the body, promoting positive gut health and quicker healing time.

Stress management is important as our body's reaction to stress can reduce our immune system's ability to fight disease. When we don't deal with our stress levels in a healthy manner, our bodies continue to produce the hormone cortisol, decreasing our response to diseases. Dealing with stress will be different for each person. Some people may need to take some time off from work to introspect, and others may find that reading a book or journaling will decrease their stress levels — it is all based on personal preference. Many people have reported that joining a meditation or yoga class will teach mechanisms that change your mindset from one of worry and stress to one of relaxation and contentment. Stress alleviation can be tough, presenting the possibility of evoking memories from the past that you weren't ready to deal with yet. This is why it is vital to speak to a professional, if you cannot find any adequate ways to relieve your stress on your own.

STEP 4: MINIMIZE TOXICITY

As humans, we communicate on a regular basis with a whole variety of different environments. Many work in areas where chemical toxicants form part of their job line, whether they are working in pest control, agriculture, or in factories. But what impact does this have on our body? How are these toxins affecting our health in the gut? Chemical toxins are a large category of environmental substances that influence our health. They have the ability to cause indefinite harm to our bodies if not monitored. Examples of these toxins include aluminium hydroxide, silicone breast implants, tobacco, glyphosate, and bisphenol A, as well as environmental toxins including heavy metals that provide a large toxic potential to the body and gut. Examples include oral lead from a root canal or a cinnabar that directly affects your liver and kidney tissue (don't worry, it is reversible). By reducing exposure, you reduce the overall toxic load on the body. Remember, environmental toxins plus a leaky gut can lead to chronic issues that will not be resolved. This is why it is important to recognize the toxins we are exposing ourselves to daily. It isn't just our diet that results in an unhealthy gut.

The toxicity of certain substances has a direct impact on our cognitive abilities. This is even more so when one deals with neurotoxins. Here are some common examples of neuro-toxins that have the potential to cause mental changes:

At least 200 chemicals have been identified as potentially neurotoxic in humans, and over 1,000 have been shown to be neurotoxic in animals, including:

- Research shows that **PBDE flame retardants** have a causal association with poorer concentration and lower scores in a large amount of childhood developmental and behavioral tests. This may ultimately result in the development of ADD or ADHD as time progresses, with the extra risk of the child needing to avoid mainstream schooling due to impaired childhood development.

- **Heavy metals, including that of lead and manganese**, have been shown to impair intelligence. With decreased levels of exposure and quick removal of the heavy metal, the degree of impaired function can be reversed. However, the effects will remain permanent if not removed.

- **Phthalates** have the potential to impair physical coordination and reduce scores in a range of behavioral tests. The effects of phthalates are said to target boys more. This may be due to the binding potential to cells within the male reproductive organs, decreasing the levels of circulating testosterone. Physically, it was noted that boys who have been exposed to phthalates showed a decreased level of physical and masculine play when compared to their classmates.

- The exposure to **air pollution** has been said to accelerate the rate at which adults experience their age-related cognitive decline. Research conducted has attributed that living in specific countries resulted in cognitive decline based on the degree and extent of air pollution that is experienced.

- A wide variety of **pesticides** are considered to increase the risk of Parkinson's disease and impair early mental development. This early mental development is characterized by the effect of one's working memory, intelligence, and ability to reason.

- **BPA** is said to affect the regulation of children's behavior. In girls, it targets emotional exacerbation, while in boys, there may be more feminine or sensitive behavior present.

STEP 5: IMPROVE DIET AND LIFESTYLE

When improving your diet, I suggest eliminating gluten, dairy, sugar, soy, corn, and all artificial preservatives. The reasons for these eliminations have all been discussed in the book and extend from GMOs not containing sufficient nutrients to foods' impact on organs in our body (e.g., soy causing our thyroid to not bind well to iodine, as well as it negatively affecting men). Living a healthy lifestyle is more than just altering your diet. One needs to always take into consideration what impact certain actions are having on your body. This could mean staying up at night to watch the next episode of your favorite series, rather than climbing into bed and getting a full eight hours of sleep. Improving your lifestyle is always better when you are doing it with someone else. Get yourself an accountability partner, and motivate and encourage each other to always make the healthiest decision possible. Remember, you are human. Make sure to remind yourself what you're working toward every day. Those reminders could be words of encouragement on your bathroom mirror or a picture board of your goals in your closet. If you happen to veer off course, that's okay, just make sure you have systems in place to get you back on track.

Some of this information seems redundant and trivial, however, it's repetition that creates a new learned pattern.

The more you hear the information, the higher likelihood it will make an impressionable effect on your health. My pathology teacher, the most difficult class I've ever taken, always said, "repetition is the mother of academia". He ensured the information was instilled into our brains. Now, it is my turn to instill in you the knowledge of how you can resolve your health issues and create a life not plagued by health concerns.

LEAVE A 1-CLICK REVIEW!

I would be incredibly thankful if you could just take 60 seconds to write a brief review on Amazon, even if it's just a few sentences.

Click Here to leave a quick review

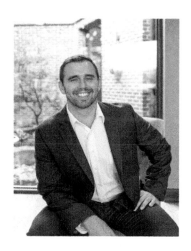

If you would like some help from me implementing strategies to help you with your health issues, then I'd like to invite you to speak with me personally.

You can work with me personally or look at my online health coaching course that gives you all the tools you need to thrive rather than merely survive.

Head over to: https://www.stronghealthplan.com/casestudy

There will be a short video and application about your health or what you need help with. (So we can review them before the call).

Answer the questions, and on the next page, you'll see a calendar with a list of available dates and times for your call. Pick the one that works best for you.

Once you have booked your time, the confirmation page will have some instructions on how to prepare for the call. Please review them thoroughly. Watch the video that breaks down what it looks like to work with me. Review the case studies from my clients. That way, when you get on the call, you will already have quite a few of your questions answered.

Once on the call, I will take a look at what you are doing, identify the problems you are having, and see if I can help. If I can help, I will show you what it looks like to work with me. You can then decide if you want to become one of my clients or not.

No pressure, but either way, you will get a lot of clarity out of this call. Visit https://www.stronghealthplan.com/casestudy to book your call today!

CONCLUSION

Gut health is an important topic in the discussion of progress toward better health. We have become so unaware of our environment, including what we feed our bodies, that it is no wonder that there are so many instances of poor gut health. The main aim of this book was to make you aware of factors that contribute to an unhealthy gut, the implications it can have on your current conditions and diseases, and how having good gut health can ultimately dictate the degree of productivity you experience on a daily basis. When we don't have good gut health, it is easy to spiral into depression, anxiety, and low self-confidence. We beat ourselves up because we aren't able to accomplish our goals. However, what we don't realize is that it wasn't because we weren't mentally prepared to do so, it's because we have not correctly treated our bodies. As soon as you start making changes that benefit your body, you will begin to realize your full mental capabilities.

Knowledge is necessary for us to effectively understand the foundation of gut health. What we should and should not eat, habits that we should try to unlearn (like saying no to receipts to reduce BPA exposure), and knowing how foods affect us are all a part of your health journey. We need to understand how our body handles inflammation and what an unhealthy gut does to our organs. Only once we understand the importance and seriousness of this can we appreciate the benefits that being healthy offers us.

The importance of nutrient supplementation has been a topic of avoidance for many years. Many do not feel the justification of using them because they haven't been 'medically' advertised and approved. However, I am hoping that this book has changed your mind. As a doctor, I have seen the positive impact that supplementation can have on the human body. Supplements have taken my patients from feeling ill and dealing with symptoms every other week to going months without having any issues. Their productivity increased, they no longer felt confined to their own bubble, and they felt like they were finally capable of pursuing their dreams. This is why supplementation is so important. It allows us to feed our body what it needs without needing to go out of our way to eat specific foods.

The strategic approach of this book was to encourage and motivate you to overcome your health problems. I have shown you how to take your problem with your gut and fix it with tried and tested solutions. This book has been your step-by-step guide on how to address your health issues. Your gut issues will affect your health, but they will be overcome after you follow the strategies in this book.

My plan was not to tell you that your gut was unhealthy, to give you a diet plan, and then send you on your way. I wanted you to understand what could happen to your gut, how

these conditions can make you feel, how to spot their development, and, most importantly, how you can go about fixing them. We spoke about the most common conditions ranging from SIBO to celiac disease; we even gave you some recipes to ensure that your gut health is always at the forefront of your dietary decisions, no matter what condition you have. I gave you all of this information so you can understand the gut and become an advocate for those that may be suffering from one of the conditions mentioned above.

You need to know how to protect your body against illness, whether by including prebiotics, probiotics, and high-fiber foods in your diet, or by ensuring you get at least a half hour of cardio exercise per day. Our lives become busy, and sometimes we discount the effect that a 30-minute exercise routine coupled with a good diet can have on our bodies. Find a group of people to exercise with and let them hold you accountable. The extent and feeling of peer support is unmatched.

Diet and gut health are not the only facets that need to be taken into consideration when creating a healthy and well-balanced lifestyle, though. We need to learn how to deal with our stress, how to avoid specific environments that are detrimental to our health, and how to make time for the activities that we enjoy. Your journey in becoming the best person you can be does not stop here. Use this book as the motivation to make your dreams a reality. Read this book as many times as you need until what you envision becomes your reality.

You read this book because you have been struggling with your health for a long time. You have experienced issues such as chronic fatigue, weight gain, pain, bloating, gas, acne, insomnia, depression, and anxiety. These have all prevented you from enjoying your life and have almost certainly made you feel more insecure. You sought out an answer to your problems, and I really hope this book offered them. One of my main goals was to establish a newfound sense of self-confidence in you that allows you to believe that you are capable of making these changes that result in a healthy gut.

"Old habits die hard" and "You are what you eat" are now a thing of the past. Remember, if you stay on your current path, you may likely develop a chronic disease down the line. By choosing to read this book, you took the first step against preventing this from happening, and your health is the most valuable asset you can invest in. Time to put in the work.

REFERENCES

Adjuvants help vaccines work better. (2019). Centers For Disease Control And Prevention. https://www.cdc.gov/vaccinesafety/concerns/adjuvants.html

Allaire, J., & Crowley, S. (2018, October 14). *The Gastrointestinal Barrier.* Colostate.Edu.

http://www.vivo.colostate.edu/hbooks/pathphys/digestion/stomach/gibarrier.html

Bahls, C. (2017, June 21). *11 Foods to Avoid During Digestive Problems and Disorders | Everyday Health.* EverydayHealth.Com. https://www.everydayhealth.com/digestive-health/diet/foods-to-avoid-during-digestive-problems/

Blood, B. (2019, April 28). *What is Celiac Disease?* Celiac Disease Foundation. https://celiac.org/about-celiac-disease/

what-is-celiac-disease/#:~:text=Celiac%20disease%
20is%20a%20serious

Breus, M. (2019, December 5). *The Connection Between Sugar and Your Gut. Psychology* Today. https://www. psychologytoday.com/za/blog/sleep-newzzz/201912/the-connection-between-sugar-and-your-gut

Bures, J. (2010). *Small intestinal bacterial overgrowth syndrome.* World Journal of Gastroenterology, 16(24), 2978. https://doi.org/10.3748/wjg.v16.i24.2978

Campos, M. (2017, September 22). *Leaky gut: What is it, and what does it mean for you?W* - Harvard Health Blog. Harvard Health Blog. https://www.health.harvard.edu/blog/leaky-gut-what-is-it-and-what-does-it-mean-for-you-2017092212451

Chavostie, C. (2019, May 28). *10 research-backed ways to improve gut health.* Www.Medicalnewstoday.Com. https://www.medicalnewstoday.com/articles/325293#reduce-stress

Cohut, M. (2019, October 23). *Common drugs may alter gut bacteria and increase health risks.* Www.Medicalnewstoday.Com. https://www.medicalnewstoday.com/articles/326766#18-common-drugs-impact-the-gut

Conlon, M., & Bird, A. (2014). *The Impact of Diet and Lifestyle on Gut Microbiota and Human Health.* Nutrients, 7(1), 17–44. https://doi.org/10.3390/nu7010017

Coyle, D. (2017, June 17). *8 Surprising Things That Harm Your Gut Bacteria.* Healthline. https://www.healthline.com/nutrition/8-things-that-harm-gut-bacteria#section6

Cummings, J. H. (1984). *Cellulose and the human gut.* Gut, 25(8), 805–810. https://doi.org/10.1136/gut.25.8.805

Detox: organs of elimination. (2016, December 7). In:Spa Retreats. https://www.inspa-retreats.com/latest-news/detox/detox-organs-of-elimination/#:~:text=Skin%3A%20The%20skin%20(your%20body

Dix, M. (2020, March 26). *7 Signs of an Unhealthy Gut and 7 Ways to Improve Gut Health.* Healthline. https://www.healthline.com/health/gut-health#treatment

Environmental Working Group. (2019a). *Clean FifteenTM Conventional Produce with the Least Pesticides.* Ewg.Org. https://www.ewg.org/foodnews/clean-fifteen.php

Environmental Working Group. (2019b). *Dirty DozenTM Fruits and Vegetables with the Most Pesticides.* Ewg.Org. https://www.ewg.org/foodnews/dirty-dozen.php

Eske, J. (2019, August 21). *Leaky gut syndrome: What it is, symptoms, and treatments.* Www.Medicalnewstoday.Com.

https://www.medicalnewstoday.com/articles/
326117#causes-and-risk-factors

Gastroesophageal Reflux Disease | AAAAI. (2019). *The American Academy of Allergy, Asthma & Immunology.* https://www.aaaai.org/conditions-and-treatments/related-conditions/gastroesophageal-reflux-disease#:~:text=Gas-troesophageal%20Reflux%20Disease%20(G ERD)%20is

Gluten-free diet: What's allowed, what's not. (2017, April 12). Mayo Clinic. https://www.mayoclinic.org/healthy-lifestyle/nutrition-and-healthy-eating/in-depth/gluten-free-diet/art-20048530

Groves, M., & Link, R. (2020, June 11). *Is Soy Good or Bad for Your Health?* Healthline. https://www.healthline.com/nutrition/soy-good-or-bad#bottom-line

Gujral, N. (2012). *Celiac disease: Prevalence, diagnosis, pathogenesis and treatment.* World Journal of Gastroenterology, 18(42), 6036. https://doi.org/10.3748/wjg.v18.i42.6036

Harvard Health Publishing. (2018, November 7). *Foods that fight inflammation - Harvard Health.* Harvard Health; Harvard Health. https://www.health.harvard.edu/staying-healthy/foods-that-fight-inflammation

Herbella, F. A. (2010). *Gastroesophageal reflux disease: From pathophysiology to treatment.* World Journal of Gastroenterology, 16(30), 3745. https://doi.org/10.3748/wjg.v16.i30.3745

Hoffman, R. (2016, July 1). *The 7 best supplements for GERD sufferers.* Drhoffman.com. https://drhoffman.com/article/the-7-best-supplements-for-gerd-sufferers/

Irritable bowel syndrome - Symptoms and causes. (2019, May 17). Mayo Clinic. https://www.mayoclinic.org/diseases-conditions/irritable-bowel-syndrome/symptoms-causes/syc-20360016#:~:text=Irritable%20bowel%20syndrome%20(IBS)%20is

Madormo, C. (2019, February 1). *SIBO: Symptoms, Treatment, Diet, and More.* Healthline. https://www.healthline.com/health/sibo#treatment

Mayer, E. A., Tillisch, K., & Gupta, A. (2015). *Gut/brain axis and the microbiota. Journal of Clinical Investigation,* 125(3), 926–938. https://doi.org/10.1172/jci76304

Meyer, J., & Michalke, K. (2008, April 18). *The Role of Metals in Gut Dysbiosis.* Www.Dr-Jacques-Imbeau.Com. http://www.dr-jacques-imbeau.com/metalsgutdysbiosis.html

Mu, Q., Kirby, J., Reilly, C. M., & Luo, X. M. (2017). *Leaky Gut As a Danger Signal for Autoimmune Diseases.* Frontiers in Immunology, 8. https://doi.org/10.3389/fimmu.2017.00598

Pick, M., OB/GYN, & NP. (2018, July 22). *BPA Health Effects On Your Gut – Is It Hazardous?* Marcelle Pick, OB/GYN NP. https://marcellepick.com/bpa-health-effects-on-your-gut/

Pizzorno, J. (2014). *Toxins From the Gut.* Integrative Medicine: A Clinician's Journal, 13(6), 8–11. https://www.ncbi.nlm.nih.gov/pmc/articles/PMC4566437/

Publishing, H. H. (2019, April 12). *The gut-brain connection.* Harvard Health. https://www.health.harvard.edu/diseases-and-conditions/the-gut-brain-connection#:~:text=A%20troubled%20intestine%20can%20send

Qin, H.-Y. (2014). *Impact of psychological stress on irritable bowel syndrome.* World Journal of Gastroenterology, 20(39), 14126. https://doi.org/10.3748/wjg.v20.i39.14126

Recipes for SIBO. (2019, October 22). Eat! Gluten-Free. https://celiac.org/eat-gluten-free/recipes/berry-jar-muffins/

Rueda-Ruzafa, L., Cruz, F., Roman, P., & Cardona, D. (2019). *Gut microbiota and neurological effects of glyphosate.* NeuroToxicology, 75, 1–8. https://doi.org/10.1016/j.neuro.2019.08.006

Shi, Z. (2019). *Gut Microbiota: An Important Link between Western Diet and Chronic Diseases.* Nutrients, 11(10), 2287. https://doi.org/10.3390/nu11102287

Tilg, H., & Kaser, A. (2011). *Gut microbiome, obesity, and metabolic dysfunction.* Journal of Clinical Investigation, 121(6), 2126–2132. https://doi.org/10.1172/jci58109

Volta, U. (2018). *Symptoms of Celiac Disease | Celiac Disease Foundation.* Celiac Disease Foundation; Celiac. https://celiac.org/about-celiac-disease/symptoms-of-celiac-disease/

Watson, S. (2015, July 22). *Autoimmune Diseases: Types, Symptoms, Causes, and More. Healthline;* Healthline Media. https://www.healthline.com/health/autoimmune-disorders#symptoms

Whitehead, W. E., Crowell, M. D., Robinson, J. C., Heller, B. R., & Schuster, M. M. (1992). *Effects of stressful life events on bowel symptoms: subjects with irritable bowel syndrome compared with subjects without bowel dysfunction.* Gut, 33(6), 825–830. https://doi.org/10.1136/gut.33.6.825